Administration
of
Imaging
Pharmaceuticals

Administration of Imaging Pharmaceuticals

Marianne Tortorici, Ed.D., ARRT(R)

Professor
Department of Radiological Sciences
University of Nevada, Las Vegas
Las Vegas, Nevada

W.B. SAUNDERS COMPANY
A Division of Harcourt Brace & Company
Philadelphia   London   Toronto
Montreal   Sydney   Tokyo

W.B. SAUNDERS COMPANY
A Division of Harcourt Brace & Company

The Curtis Center
Independence Square West
Philadelphia, Pennsylvania 19106

Library of Congress Cataloging-in-Publication Data

Administration of imaging pharmaceuticals/[edited by]
Marianne Tortorici.—1st ed.
 p. cm.
 ISBN 0–7216–4813–4
 1. Radiopharmaceuticals. 2. Contrast media. I. Tortorici,
Marianne R.
 [DNLM: 1. Diagnostic Imaging—methods. 2. Diagnosis,
Radioisotope. 3. Contrast Media. WN 180 I305 1996]
RM852.I47 1996
616.07′575—dc20
DNLM/DLC   96–6051

ADMINISTRATION OF IMAGING PHARMACEUTICALS   ISBN 0–7216–4813–4

Last digit is the print number: 9   8   7   6   5   4   3   2   1

In Memory

This text is dedicated to
Dr. Hiram Morris Hunt,
who for 15 years served as my mentor.
He willingly offered me his wisdom,
unselfishly assisted me in writing my
dissertation, and coauthored two
laboratory manuals with me.
The only reimbursement he asked of me
was to promise to share my knowledge
and experience with others.
This text is written as one means of
fulfilling that promise.

Contributors

Joseph R. Bittengle, M.Ed., ARRT(R)
Department of Radiologic Technology
University of Arkansas for Medical Sciences
Little Rock, Arkansas
Contrast Media; Preventive Care and Emergency Response to Contrast Media

Donna C. Davis, M.Ed., ARRT(R)(CV)
Department of Radiologic Technology
University of Arkansas for Medical Sciences
Little Rock, Arkansas
Contrast Media; Preventive Care and Emergency Response to Contrast Media

Ann Obergfell, J.D., ARRT(R)
University of Louisville
Radiologic Technology Program
Louisville, Kentucky
Legal Opinion: Pro

Milton Schwartzberg, J.D.
Boston, Massachusetts
Legal Opinion: Con

Preface

This text is designed as a teaching tool for imaging technologists who elect to inject drugs. In light of the controversy surrounding whether technologists should inject, this text provides the reader with two legal opinions on the subject: one in support of venipuncture and one against the practice of venous injection of drugs by registered technologists. Both opinions are written by attorneys. In states that have no laws prohibiting the technologist from injecting, the decision as to whether to administer drugs to patients rests with the individual technologist. For those technologists assuming the responsibilty of injection, this text provides a background in pharmacology overview, drug measurements and dose calculation, contrast media, preventive care and emergency response to contrast media reactions, precautions when mixing contrast media or radiopharmaceuticals with other drugs, parenteral injection techniques, and record keeping.

It should be noted that pharmacology is a very complex and extensive topic. This text provides a summary of the areas of pharmacology most applicable to the technologist. Also, the types of parenteral injection techniques presented are limited to those a technologist is most apt to use.

It is strongly recommended that this text be used in conjunction with formal education by a qualified instructor. Additionally, it is strongly recommended that the textbook instruction be supplemented with appropriately supervised practical experience.

MARIANNE TORTORICI, Ed.D., ARRT(R)

Acknowledgments

This text was completed with the assistance of several people and companies. Many are students and colleagues whom I met over the years whose belief in me and words of encouragement provided me with the faith and persistence I needed to pursue such a large venture as writing a text.

I would also like to thank Lance Nicholls and Mary Ricci for their assistance in the secretarial work associated with the development of the manuscript, which included, but was not limited to, correspondence, obtaining permission forms, and copying manuscript pages.

I am grateful to Mr. Michael Bloyd, R.N., ARRT(R), and Colleen Keller, R.N., Ph.D., for their patience and constructive comments in reviewing the manuscript material.

Additionally, I would like to express my appreciation to Lisa Biello, Vice President and Editor-in-Chief, Health-Related Professions, at the W.B. Saunders Company, for her assistance and invaluable guidance in the development of this text. I am especially grateful for her words of encouragement and understanding during times of stress.

Several companies provided charts, tables, or photographs, used throughout this text. I would like to thank the F.A. Davis Company and the J.B. Lippincott Company for allowing the reproduction of their material.

Contents

Introduction

1

Development of the Allied Health
  Concept
Evolution of Radiologic Technology
  Education
Scope of Practice
Current Educational Standards for
  Technologists
Position of the States on
  Venipuncture

DEVELOPMENT OF THE ALLIED HEALTH CONCEPT

Humans have been practicing medicine since ancient times. From primitive times to about the 18th century, the practice of medicine was based on religion and magic. Disease was thought to be caused by gods or spirits. During these times, the most common treatments for disease included suckling, fumigating, bleeding, steam baths, and herbs. However, in ancient China, disease was treated by nourishing the body, medication, and acupuncture. During the Dark Ages, exorcism, images of saints, the supernatural, and superstition were the tools to treat disease. It wasn't until the Renaissance that medical practices became more scientifically oriented. For example, Harvey described the closed circulatory system, da Vinci drew meticulous anatomic diagrams, and Huygens developed the centigrade system.

Advancements in medicine continued in the 18th century with such milestones as Jenner's discovery of a smallpox vaccination, Hales' ability to measure blood pressure and demonstrate the dynamics of blood circulation, and Hunter's method of closing off aneurysms. By the end of the 19th century, the basis for much of modern medicine was established, which included Lister's discovery of bacteria, Pasteur's development of aseptic technique, Mendel's establishment of his theory on genetics, and Roentgen's discovery of x-rays.

By the 20th century, the advent of these new technologic discoveries led to a rapid increase in the demands for health care services. The one-to-one interaction between doctor and patient and physician visits to patients' homes became things of the past. New technologies became so complex that their proper operation required specially trained personnel. As these health technologies developed their own autonomy, the people within the specific fields began to form their own professional societies.

Professional allied health societies evolved for a number of reasons. Some of the reasons were to prevent incompetent people from practicing, to standardize the training of personnel, to reduce the competition in the job market, and to protect the individual's position. One major outcome of the professional societies was the establishment of standards of practice based on minimum educational requirements, which often culminate in a person's having to pass a registry or certification examination (or both) in order to practice.

Originally, professional societies were responsible for the development and implementation of registries and standards for certification. As time progressed, the American Medical Association (AMA) became involved in accrediting allied health education programs. Eventually, to become eligible to write a specific registry or to qualify for certification, allied health personnel had to graduate from a school accredited by the AMA. Until 1992, school accreditation was contingent on an institution complying with the "Essentials" or guidelines established by the AMA through the Committee on Allied Health Education and Accreditation

(CAHEA) and its various review committees. In 1992, the AMA dissolved CAHEA. As of this writing, no other organization has replaced CAHEA. However, the various joint review committees once associated with CAHEA still exist. These committees continue to review schools for accreditation. The last directory published by the AMA (1994–1995), which lists accredited allied health schools, identified approximately 30 different allied health disciplines (Table 1–1). Each field is autonomous in matters of training, certifying, and setting standards for professional practice. The field of radiologic technology is one of the disciplines recognized by the AMA.

TABLE 1–1

Allied Health Fields Identified by the AMA

Allied Health Discipline	Occupational Title
Anesthesiology Assistant	Anesthesiologist's Assistant
Athletic Training	Athletic Trainer
Blood Bank Technology	Specialist in blood bank technology
Cardiovascular Technology	Cardiovascular Technologist
Cytotechnology	Cytotechnologist
Diagnostic Medical Sonography	Diagnostic Medical Sonographer
Electroneurodiagnostic Technology	Electroneurodiagnostic Technologist
Emergency Medical Services	Emergency Medical Technician—Paramedic
Medical Assisting	Medical Assistant
Medical Illustration	Medical Illustrator
Medical Laboratory Technology	Histologic Technician
	Histologic Technologist
	Medical Laboratory Technician (Associate's Degree)
	Medical Laboratory Technician (Certificate)
	Medical Technologist
Medical Record Administration (Health Information Administration)	Medical Record Administrator (Health Information Administrator)
	Medical Record Technician (Health Information Technician)
Nuclear Medicine Technology	Nuclear Medicine Technologist
Occupational Therapy	Occupational Therapy Assistant
	Occupational Therapist
Ophthalmic Medical Technology	Ophthalmic Medical Technician
	Ophthalmic Medical Technologist
Perfusion	Perfusionist
Physician Assistant Practice	Physician Assistant
	Surgeon Assistant
Radiologic Technology	Radiation Therapy Technologist
	Radiographer
Respiratory Therapy	Respiratory Therapist
	Respiratory Therapy Technician
Surgical Technology	Surgical Technologist

EVOLUTION OF RADIOLOGIC TECHNOLOGY EDUCATION

Radiologic technology began developing its autonomy in the United States through the establishment of a national registry for radiographers (radiologic technologists) in 1922. The registry was called the American Registry of Radiologic Technicians and was supported by the Radiological Society of North America (the American College of Radiology replaced the Radiological Society of North America in 1944) and the American Roentgen Ray Society. Additional cooperation for the establishment of a registry came from the Canadian Association of Radiologists and the American Society of X-ray Technicians (forerunner of the American Society of Radiologic Technologists, or ASRT). Forty years after the founding of the American Registry of Radiologic Technicians, the name of the organization changed to the American Registry of Radiologic Technologists (ARRT). Certification was provided in the area of nuclear medicine in 1963. Radiation therapy certification began in 1964. In 1977, the term *radiographer* was adopted to replace "x-ray technologist."

The population of radiologic technologists (radiography, radiation therapy, and nuclear medicine) has substantially increased since 1922 and is continuing to grow at a rapid pace. For example, in 1962, there were approximately 31,000 registered radiologic technologists. Ten years later, the number of registered radiologic technologists had more than doubled (to approximately 65,000). By 1992, the number of registered technologists had reached approximately 180,000.

Although CAHEA accredited only four occupational fields in the diagnostic imaging and therapeutic areas (radiography, nuclear medicine, radiation therapy, and sonography), the ARRT offers certification in mammography, cardiovascular intervention technology, computed radiography, and magnetic resonance imaging. Discussion is underway to determine if the areas of quality assurance, administration, and education should offer a certification.

SCOPE OF PRACTICE

A common method used to define an occupational scope of practice is task analysis. Task analysis involves the identification of tasks associated with a specific job. Several methods are used to perform a task analysis. The ASRT and the ARRT have used task analysis to develop educator's curriculum guides and certification examinations, respectively. A list of all the tasks associated with the three fields of radiologic technology is beyond the scope of this text. However, because this text is concerned with the administration of drugs, a brief discussion on venipuncture as an appropriate task within the scope of practice of a technologist is in order.

Prior to discussing scope of practice, it should be noted that "scope of practice" is used loosely in this chapter and in no way is intended to refer to its legal definition. The reader is referred to Chapters 2 and 3 on the pros and cons of legal opinion for specific information on a legal interpretation of scope of practice.

The Joint Review Committee on Education in Radiologic Technology (JRCERT) is the agency primarily responsible for accrediting educational programs in radiography and radiation therapy. The Joint Review Committee on Nuclear Medicine (JRCNM) is the agency primarily responsible for accrediting educational programs in nuclear medicine. These agencies establish the criteria that educational institutions must meet to maintain accreditation. The criteria are written in a booklet containing guidelines for accreditation and are referred to as the "Essentials." As of this writing, the JRCNM Essentials, under "DESCRIPTION OF THE PROFESSION, B. Technical Skills, no. 2," states:

Prepare and administer radiopharmaceuticals, where permitted, to patients by intravenous, intramuscular, subcutaneous and oral methods.

Also, in Section III, Curriculum B, supervised clinical education, no. 4 of the JRCNM states:

Preparing, calculating, identifying, administering (where permitted), and disposing of radiopharmaceuticals.

Therefore, the JRCNM has identified drug administration and venipuncture as a part of a nuclear medicine technologist's scope of practice. However, the JRCERT Essentials do not identify the administration of pharmaceuticals or venipuncture as a part of the tasks to be performed by radiographers and radiation therapists. It should be noted that the JRCNM and JRCERT use the ASRT curriculum guides to develop the guidelines and Essentials for educational programs. In 1991, the ASRT approved the incorporation of venipuncture as part of the jobs of radiographers and radiation therapists. It is anticipated that the JRCERT will continue its policy of using the ASRT curriculum guide to develop the Essentials. Therefore, the JRCERT probably will add venipuncture to its list of minimum educational requirements for radiographers and radiation therapists in its next revision of the Essentials.

Additional support for the administration of drugs and venipuncture as a part of the job descriptions of radiographers and radiation therapists is given by the American College of Radiology's (ACR) 1987 resolution no. 27. In this resolution, the ACR stated that it "approves of the injection of contrast material and diagnostic levels of radiopharmaceutical by certified and/or licensed radiologic technologists . . .".

Currently, whether or not radiologic technologists should be responsible for the venous administration of drugs is the subject of much debate.

CURRENT EDUCATIONAL STANDARDS FOR TECHNOLOGISTS

Although the ARRT no longer recognizes only one national accrediting agency for radiography, radiation therapy, and nuclear medicine, the various joint review committees are still the primary organization assuming that position. It is assumed that the standards established over the years by the joint review committees will continue to serve as the minimum standards of education for technologists in the near future. As such, persons graduating from a school of radiography accredited by a joint review committee must have a minimum of 2 years of postsecondary education. Nuclear medicine technologists must have at least 1 year of postsecondary education and often need additional qualifications, such as being a radiographer, prior to being admitted to a nuclear medicine program. In the year 2000, radiation therapists will have to have a bachelor's degree to enter a radiation therapy program. All of these disciplines require courses in patient care and intense clinical experience. Radiographers receive additional education in contrast media, and nuclear medicine technologists are educated in radiopharmaceuticals and their administration.

POSITION OF THE STATES ON VENIPUNCTURE

A national survey conducted in 1993 by Tortorici and MacDonald summarized the official position of the radiation control office of 50 states and the District of Columbia relative to technologists injecting contrast medium, radiopharmaceuticals, or other drugs. The objective of the survey was to determine which states had a state statute, rule, or regulation relevant to parenteral injection of drugs by technologists. Of the 49 states responding to the questionnaire, 26 states had some form of licensure. However, not all modalities were listed under state statutes. Only 17 states (34.7%) had a licensure or certification in all three modalities. Five additional states (10.2%) had a licensure or certificate requirement in radiography and radiation therapy, but not nuclear medicine. Four other states (8.2%) required a license or certification in radiography only. Licensure for nuclear medicine only was required in two states. The remaining 23 states did not have licensure or certification.

The bills reviewed by Tortorici and MacDonald revealed that only California, Illinois, Montana, New Jersey, New York, and Utah had any kind of statement relative to technologists performing venipuncture. All of these states, with the exception of New Jersey, provided regulations authorizing the nuclear medicine technologist to administer contrast media or other drugs. California and New York specifically prohibited radiographers and therapists from performing venipuncture. New Jersey prohibits radiographers and radiation therapist technologists from performing venipuncture and from injecting contrast media or other drugs.

BIBLIOGRAPHY

Allied health education directory 1994–1995, 22nd edition. Committee on Allied Health Accreditation and Education, Chicago, 1994.

American registry of radiologic technologists, the first fifty (1922–1972). American Registry of Radiologic Technologists, Minneapolis, November 1972.

American registry of radiologic technologist's educator's handbook, 3rd edition. American Registry of Radiologic Technologists, Mendota Heights, MN, January 1990.

Bender, CE: Misinterpretation in venipuncture article [letter]. Wavelength 3(6):6, March 1992.

Bloyd, M: Venipuncture technique. 1992 American Society of Radiologic Technologists Annual Meeting, Salt Lake City, June 1992.

Hatfield, S: Venipuncture makes way into radiologic science curricula. Advance for Radiologic Science Professionals (592):5, January 13, 1992.

Essentials and guidelines of an accredited educational program for the nuclear medicine technologist. Joint Review Committee on Educational Programs in Nuclear Medicine Technology, Chicago, 1991.

Essentials and guidelines of an accredited educational program for the radiologic technologist. Joint Review Committee on Educational Programs in Radiologic Technology, 1990.

Loudin, A: Preparing for venipuncture. RT Image 4(24):1, June 17, 1991.

McTernan, EJ, and Hawkins, RO: Educating personnel for the allied health professions and services. CV Mosby, St. Louis, 1972.

Mixdorf, M, and Goldsworthy, R: The radiography essentials: an evolutionary perspective. Radiol Tech 63(6):386 July/August 1992.

Poteet, M: Venipuncture—has the time come? Wavelength 3(1):1 October 1991.

Tortorici, MR: Task analysis of special procedures radiography and computerized axial tomography technology [dissertation]. University of Houston, August 1979.

Tortorici, MR, and MacDonald, JM: RTs performing venipuncture: a survey of state regulations. Radiol Tech 64(6):368 July/August 1993.

Walters, R: Venipuncture issue makes blood boil [letter]. Wavelength 3(8):6 May 1992.

Legal Opinion: Pro

ANN OBERGFELL, J.D., ARRT(R)

2

INTRODUCTION

The changing scene in health care delivery is causing many professional organizations and accrediting agencies to reevaluate how the profession educates its members and controls admission to its ranks. The radiologic science professions are no different, as exemplified by the review and revision of the scopes of practice and the curriculum guides for each discipline.

Constantly growing and changing professions require that educational guidelines and scopes of practice reflect the activity and function of the members as part of a dynamic health care delivery system. The issues of venipuncture and administration of contrast media, radiopharmaceuticals, and related drugs are two of the primary concerns in the changing practice of the radiologic sciences. Many technologists are required to administer these pharmaceuticals, either by the physician to whom they must answer or to an administration that must streamline departments and cut the cost of potentially unnecessary personnel, such as nurses who currently, though questionably, are permitted to administer these medications.

The American Society of Radiologic Technologists has attempted to alleviate the concerns of radiologic technologists by expanding the scope of practice[1] to include venipuncture and by introducing sections on venipuncture, administration of contrast media, and pharmacology into the curriculum guide.[2]

By sanctioning technologists to administer contrast media, the profession has not only greatly expanded the role of the technologist but has increased the liability placed on radiographers and nuclear medicine technologists, the physicians who work with them, and the facilities that employ them. It is, therefore, imperative that these medical imaging professionals understand the responsibility undertaken, learn what is expected, and perform only those procedures which they are educationally qualified to undertake.

The changes in the scopes of practice and the curriculum guides are not only timely but are essential if the professions are to grow and mature in the newly emerging health care delivery system.

ONE PERSON'S OPINION

As the health care scene changes, so must the professional practice of radiographers and nuclear medicine technologists. It is time to emerge from the shadows of the physician and take a rightful place in the health care mainstream. The struggle for autonomy has been long coming; many inside and outside the profession have pledged resistance, yet, even as the arguments rage, the role of the technologist has expanded, the responsibility has increased, and the liability has extended.

For many years, radiographers in several parts of the country have been administering contrast media without appropriate education and without a real understanding of the potential consequences of their actions. The drug administration was generally ordered by a physician, yet the physician was not present, had not seen the patient, and often was not prepared to deal with a potential reaction. Many times contrast media are ordered by physicians who have no knowledge of the composition of the pharmaceutical or its contraindications. The knowledge of the physician was, and still is, in many cases limited to the resultant diagnosis of the procedure rather than the means used to obtain the desired result. The ramifications of the practice of administering pharmaceuticals are far reaching, and until recently, radiographers were performing a function that was neither sanctioned by the profession nor included in the approved educational guidelines. The practice not only endangered the patient but placed the radiographer at great risk. In the eyes of the law, although liability for adverse reactions generally rested with the physician, the radiographer was, and is, responsible for his or her own actions.

Even in light of these negative ramifications and increased liability, the radiographer is the most appropriate health care professional to perform venipuncture and administer contrast media. The radiographer is the person who prepares the room, discusses the procedure with the patient, acquires the pertinent patient history, and stays with the patient after the contrast medium has been administered. Professionally, the radiographer is trained to assess the patient and to be alert to subtle changes that may indicate a reaction. The radiographer is trained in emergency procedures and is prepared to begin cardiopulmonary resuscitation (CPR) or to follow other emergency protocols. With the addition of venipuncture and pharmacology to the curriculum, the technologist should be more than prepared to meet the demands of the expanding role in diagnostic imaging.

Likewise, the nuclear medicine technologist is the appropriate professional to administer radiopharmaceuticals. The education of nuclear medicine technologists includes radiopharmacy, radiation protection, and radiation biology, as well as patient care skills in emergency procedures, sterile technique, and injection, including venipuncture.

Some who believe a registered nurse is the correct person to inject contrast media and radiopharmaceuticals in the diagnostic imaging department need only look to the respective knowledge and skill levels to note that a nurse does not have the background in radiopharmacy, contrast media, radiation protection, and radiation biology necessary to administer these substances. Likewise, a radiologist may be able to administer the pharmaceuticals but is often not readily available in the diagnostic imaging department, or, because of time constraints, may not be able to stay in the area for an extended period post injection. Because many reactions do not occur immediately upon injection, the radiologist or nurse must stay in the area if they are to effectively respond to an adverse reaction.

INCREASED COST OF CARE

The increased cost of health care is a primary concern of every American and of the health care industry. If radiographers and nuclear medicine technologists are prohibited from performing venipuncture and administering contrast media, other health care professionals, such as nurses or physicians, will need to be present before, during, and after all contrast media and radiopharmaceuticals administrations. The radiographer or nuclear medicine technologist will likewise need to be present, because such workers are the professionals with the knowledge and skill necessary to complete the procedure.

Cross-training of nurses in the radiologic sciences would require that nurses complete all procedural, technical, and radiation courses to become competent in handling the procedural aspects of the diagnostic imaging department. Cross-training radiographers would only require education in the areas of venipuncture, contrast media administration, and pharmacology. Although nursing training could require as much as 2 years of academic preparation for such duties, the radiographer would at most require a semester or at least a current patient care course expanded to include venipuncture and contrast media administration and a pharmacology course. The new curriculum guide for radiography includes these concepts and is already set in motion in many programs across the country.

With the increasing concern over the cost of health care services, it does not seem fiscally prudent to maintain additional high-paid persons, such as nurses, in a diagnostic imaging area when the technologist—the person most qualified to administer the pharmaceutical, respond to any reactions, and complete the diagnostic procedure—is already available in the department. Health care delivery is changing, radiography education is changing, and the profession must change to meet the expanding role of radiologic science professionals in the areas of patient-focused care and cost containment.

SCOPE OF PRACTICE

A basic principle in the law that justifies and encourages the expanded role of radiographers and nuclear medicine technologists in the areas of venipuncture and administration of contrast media and radiopharmaceuticals is the *scope of practice*. The concept of scope of practice is founded in the principle of defining those activities which a person participates in during the course of employment and because of educational foundation and professional experience is prepared to perform.

If a plaintiff claims that a radiographer or nuclear medicine technologist has negligently performed an injection and has caused some injury, the plaintiff's attorney will investigate the activity surrounding the incident to determine if something had been done improperly. Part of the investigation will include an evaluation of a radiography or nuclear medicine scope of practice. Because the recently redrafted scopes of practice include venipuncture and pharmacology, the attorney will probably not try to claim that the radiographer or nuclear medicine technologist acted outside of the scope of practice. With further investigation, the attorney will try to discover if the radiographer or nuclear medicine technologist had the appropriate education and experience to perform the injection.

Therefore, it is imperative that radiographers and nuclear medicine technologists be properly trained in venipuncture technique and contrast media or radiopharmaceutical administration. It is also important that they periodically update their knowledge of contrast media or radiopharmaceuticals and that they remain current with changes in the practice and in pharmaceuticals. The American Society of Radiologic Technologists' curriculum guides for radiographers and nuclear medicine technologists are the best starting points for those who are trying to determine if they have met professional guidelines.

STANDARD OF CARE

A second and important aspect of liability centers around the concept of the standard of care. This principle in the law of negligence requires that the courts look to the degree of care that a reasonably prudent person should exercise under the same or similar circumstances. In the case of health care professionals, the standard is that the professional in question exercise the average degree of skill, care, and diligence exercised by other members of the same profession practicing in the same or similar circumstances.[3] If the answer is no, the investigation would turn on why the radiographer or nuclear medicine technologist chose to perform the test.

The current standard seems to be that in most cases, radiographers with the appropriate education and experience may perform venipuncture and administer contrast media. In 1977, an Indiana court considered the education of radiographers and determined that radiographers did not have the education necessary to determine whether the physician had selected an inappropriate means of injection for contrast media.[4] Although the court could find no evidence that a radiographer's education was adequate for determining the appropriate means of injection in 1977, it is not clear that the same decision would be reached today because of the changes in the scope of practice, the revised radiography curriculum, which includes venipuncture and contrast media administration, and the current standard of care for radiographers.

Exceptions to the current trend in the standard are found in states where radiographers are prohibited from performing venipuncture and administering contrast media by state statute or regulation. Each state is permitted to draft legislation concerning the activities of health care providers practicing within the state. Some states have indicated that only physicians, dentists, and registered nurses may perform venipuncture. Others have indicated that only physicians, dentists, pharmacists, and registered nurses may administer pharmaceuticals. Few states have adopted these guidelines, but it is important to determine whether the state in which the radiographer or nuclear medicine technologist practices has adopted such a statute or regulation. A jury in Washington state was allowed to hear the effects of a practical nurse's violation of a state statute allowing only registered nurses to perform injections. The court determined that the public policy issue underlying the ruling and the statute was that a person undertaking a task of a registered nurse must have the knowledge and skill possessed by a licensed registered nurse, the implication being that if the defendant was not a licensed registered nurse, she or he did not have the same skill and knowledge.[5]

A defendant radiographer in the same situation may be able to demonstrate that the skill and knowledge is present because of current educational guidelines and scope of practice. However, statutes that contain language limiting those who may perform a specific activity are generally construed as absolute.

Nuclear medicine technologists may run into the same problems in the administration of radiopharmaceuticals, but the educational process in nuclear medicine has included the administration of radiopharmaceuticals for a longer period of time and is therefore not as controversial. Others intimate that the chances of reaction from radiopharmaceuticals are less than with contrast media. Although this may be true, one need only look at the nature of the pharmaceutical to see the dangers inherent in both preparation and administration.

PERSONAL RESPONSIBILITY

Another basic principle in the law of negligence, which many in the radiologic sciences overlook, is that each person is responsible for his or her own actions. Placing the blame on the physician's order may be effective to a point, but it does not explain why a person has performed a procedure that he or she did not have the necessary knowledge and skill to perform. A family practice physician, although a doctor, probably does not have the skill to perform delicate brain surgery, even if ordered to do so and under the direct supervision of a neurosurgeon. The law would find this type of practice contrary to public policy and a grave breach of the duty owed to the patient.

Radiologic science professionals must take responsibility for the acts they perform in a professional capacity. To blindly follow orders without having the appropriate skills and knowledge necessary to perform a task violates the public trust and is not permitted by law.

LONG-TERM EFFECTS OF MAINTAINING THE STATUS QUO

Radiographers and nuclear medicine technologists must take responsibility for the practices that they undertake. They must understand what they are doing, why they are doing it, and how they are expected to perform. Radiographers and nuclear medicine technologists who continue on the path of least resistance by following the orders of a physician when the practice is contrary to the knowledge and skills of the radiologic science professional or when they do not possess the skills necessary to perform said task are placing not only themselves but the patient and the physician at great risk.

Allowing physicians, nurses, and legislators to determine what a radiologic science professional can and cannot, or should and should not, do in the scope of their professional practice is contrary to self-determination and places the radiologic sciences professional in the position of second-class citizens. Likewise, radiographers and nuclear medicine technologists who believe that allowing other health care professionals to dictate the practice will limit their personal liability are naive and are setting themselves up for a great fall if they are named in a medical negligence law suit.

If radiologic science professionals refuse to take on the role of a competent professional by expanding their role in venipuncture and administration of contrast media and radiopharmaceuticals, the practice may be taken from them. Others may be trained in these areas, taking a part of the practice that should rightfully be in the hands of radiographers and nuclear medicine technologists.

If technologists continue to perform venipuncture and contrast media administration without the necessary and appropriate knowledge and skill as required by the new professional guidelines and expanded scope of practice, they are placing themselves at risk for claims of negligent professional practice. Hiding behind the coattails of a physician will not exclude the radiographer from personal liability.

SUMMARY

Health care reform in the United States is a reality waiting to happen. Radiologic science professionals must maintain and upgrade the status of their discipline. By allowing it to flounder, they open up the possibility that change will occur from outside the profession. Such changes, imposed by those who do not understand the practice or the long-term effects of malpractice, are undesirable. The profession must first educate its own members and then educate the general public as to the knowledge and skill of radiographers and nuclear medicine technologists.

BIBLIOGRAPHY

1. Scope of practice for radiologic technologists. American Society of Radiologic Technologists, Albuquerque, 1993.
2. Curriculum guide for programs in radiologic technology. American Society of Radiologic Technologists, Albuquerque, 1992.
3. Black's Law Dictionary, 5th edition. West Publishing Co, St. Paul, 1979.
4. Brook v. St. John Hickeg Memorial Hospital, 368 NE2d 264 (Ind. 1977).
5. Barber v. Reinking, 411 P2d 861 (1966).

Legal Opinion: Con

MILTON SCHWARTZBERG, J.D.

3

INTRODUCTION

In initially examining the question of whether or not radiologic technologists should be permitted to perform venipuncture and administer drugs, the logical and sensible answer seems to be apparent. After all, radiologic technologists are already positioned to do so by virtue of their existing duties. Many, in fact, have long done so as a routine part of their employment, either under the directive of a physician or by custom of the medical facility.

There is no doubt that inconsistency and variation seem to be the rule relative to state laws governing this practice. Furthermore, the profession (along with all allied-health fields) is currently experiencing explosive growth and with it changes in curricula, focus, and, consequently, practice.

It is this evolutionary process in the profession, among other things, that some use to justify expansion into the field of venipuncture and the administration of pharmacological agents. After all, would this not reduce the personnel necessary to perform diagnostic procedures? Would this not, more importantly, lead to a reduction in costs as well as increase efficiency?

It is my contention that, currently, expansion of the profession into this field would be counterproductive and would actually raise health care costs as well as expose radiologic technologists to the needless risk of further legal liability. Additionally, until state laws and university curricula are consistent nationwide, radiologic technologists would be ill advised to expand into this area.

I will more closely examine the foregoing in this chapter. Constraints on length prevent me from discussing each and every facet of this controversial question. I will, therefore, limit my discussion to the areas that I feel are most influential in addressing this critical question.

COST OF HEALTH CARE

As the demands on the profession increase, so will the diversity of pressures it faces. One of these is to specifically focus on cost reduction in the delivery of services. This is to be performed within the larger context of the overall containment of health care costs.

The costs of medical care are enormous, both to individuals and to society, and they continue to increase. Over the last 15 years, the proportion of the gross national product used to finance health care has risen from 5.9% to 14%. Many factors contribute to this situation: slow growth of the gross national product, general economic inflation, advances in technology, population growth, real price increases for services, administrative costs, malpractice expenses, and an aging population.

The proportion of health care expenditures paid by federal sources has risen rapidly in recent years, draining resources for education, social programs, and other public needs. In the private sector, the relative burden has shifted from an individual-payor emphasis to a greater proportion of expenditures covered by employer-paid health insurance benefits. According to O'Neill, "Controlling costs has become a priority. In response to the ever increasing costs of health care, both the private and public sectors have developed a host of new approaches aimed at containing the rate of growth. . . ."[1]

The issue of health care costs has international implications as well. The cost of manufactured goods such as automobiles and computers is largely affected by the amount of worker health care costs. As these costs rise, so do the product prices, and the products become less competitive in the international marketplace at a time when our country is meeting its highest levels of worldwide competition ever.

On the domestic scene, the largest employer of workers in the country, small businesses, has recently been hit with record numbers of bankruptcies. These were caused in large part by increased worker health care costs. Many businesses have chosen to relocate all or part of their operations overseas to avoid this expense. Either way, rising health care costs affect virtually everyone negatively.

Most employers are now passing an ever-increasing proportion of their health care costs to their employees. This inevitably reduces employee disposable income in the short term and standard of living in the long term. We have often heard that the so-called "baby boomer" generation, and especially their children, cannot maintain the standard of living that their parents enjoyed (and that they themselves experienced during their formative years in the 1950s and 1960s). Although there are myriad reasons for this downward spiral in the standard of living (especially in the blue collar occupations), health care costs, especially in the last 15 years, are a major culprit.

Because every man, woman, and child is affected by both the need for medical services and their actual and "passed-on" costs, this has become a hot political issue. The fact that health care costs have consistently outpaced inflation made this issue a centerpiece of the 1992 presidential campaign. Indeed, all the major candidates promised overhaul of the health care delivery system as well as cost containment. President Clinton promised a revamped health care systemic plan within the "first one hundred days" of his administration. The complexity of this issue soon overwhelmed those assigned to deal with it. The only certainty appears that our health care system is undergoing fundamental change. This period of transition is likely to last for years. Because of both its high cost and high public demand, the restructuring of the health care system is likely to be controversial for years to come. Certainly, containment of health care costs is a goal that nearly all Americans would welcome.

In light of the foregoing, we must examine the role of the technologist in lowering, or at least containing, health care costs. Again, questions arise concerning venipuncture and the administration of drugs:

1. Is it not cost effective to allow the technologist to perform these functions in place of more highly compensated physicians and nurses?

2. Is not venipuncture and drug administration a natural extension of the technologist's role?
3. Would not this extension promote efficiency and, consequently, cost effectiveness?

Before these questions can be answered fully, we must examine a number of diverse issues. Among these issues are:

1. Varying educational standards and curricula throughout the country
2. Diverse licensing requirements enacted by the states
3. Varying state statutes and what activities they permit and prohibit
4. Diverse customs and practices as they affect the role of the technologist
5. Medical malpractice and its implications

LIMITING MEDICAL MALPRACTICE COSTS

Few areas of the law have been the subject of as much controversy in this country as has medical malpractice. Impassioned arguments have been made by nearly all parties involved.

Physicians and their varied professional associations have urged curbs on recovery by plaintiffs, as well as procedural hurdles, to make the entire process more cumbersome for those seeking redress. We have all heard the stories of certain medical practitioners (most notably obstetricians and surgeons) being forced to pay huge and ever-increasing amounts in medical malpractice insurance premiums. Many were forced out of practice as a result.

In response to this situation, many state legislatures enacted laws in the late 1970s and early 1980s that set up obstacles making it more difficult to institute and prosecute a medical malpractice lawsuit. These actions were met with bitter opposition from the organized trial bar. Lawyers took the position that acts of medical malpractice that had previously been ignored were now being prosecuted because of greater public awareness. Their position was that a relatively small number of doctors were responsible for the vast majority of malpractice claims. It was because the medical profession failed to police itself adequately that these "bad" doctors were able to victimize the public, often with devastating consequences. Attorneys were often criticized as the result of a few highly publicized and large contingent fee awards. Doctors maintained that these awards and exorbitant fees were the primary cause behind the ever-increasing malpractice insurance premiums. Lawyers responded by stating that the system of contingent fees permits access to the legal system for the vast majority of the public that otherwise would be unable to afford it.

Balancing the concerns of the legal and medical communities, while simultaneously acting in the public interest, puts lawmakers in a quandary. One solution enacted in Massachusetts was to place medical malpractice cases into a separate class and set up certain procedural hurdles. The purpose of these hurdles was to weed out frivolous actions and allow the more egrégious cases to proceed. Specifically, soon after a medical malpractice lawsuit is filed, the case is evaluated by a tribunal (panel).

This panel consists of a judge, lawyer (unrelated to the case), and physician whose specialty is the area of medicine involved in the suit. After hearing a presentation by each side, the tribunal deliberates the viability of the subject action. A majority of the panel would have to rule that the case is legitimate and serious and that the plaintiff's injuries were caused by the doctor's failure to meet the recognized standards of medical care and treatment then prevailing in the community for the lawsuit to proceed unimpeded. If the panel finds that the doctor had met the prevailing community medical standards and that the injuries were sustained as a result of an unavoidable or unfortunate medical outcome, the plaintiff would have to post a bond before the case would be allowed to go forward. In some instances, such a ruling would be sufficient to extinguish a case. (It should be noted that such cases were voluntarily withdrawn and not by order of the court.) In my personal experience of sitting on several medical malpractice tribunals, the injuries presented always were severe, and all panel members were unanimous in deciding to allow the case to proceed unimpeded.

However, it is noteworthy that in the vast majority of cases (believed to be as high as 80% to 90%), the eventual outcome is a finding in the defendant doctor's favor. Many theories attempt to explain this phenomenon, ranging from effective insurance company propaganda in the media to a more sophisticated (and cost-conscious) population now sitting on juries. Because most medical malpractice insurance carriers aggressively defend these cases, very few are settled before trial. Litigation, which frequently drags on for several years, is expensive. Therefore, these defendants' verdicts do not immediately translate into lower insurance premiums, although the rate of increase is significantly lower than it was in the past.

The legal theories of medical malpractice are varied and complex. It is not the purpose of this chapter to closely examine them. However, a brief overview of some of these theories will help to explain my contention that venipuncture by technologists would actually increase health care costs as opposed to the prevailing view in the radiologic technologists profession that costs would be reduced.

NEGLIGENCE

Currently, in the United States, there are two major theories of liability (or responsibility) for acts of alleged medical malpractice. The most widely employed of these is the negligence theory. As in all lawsuits, the plaintiff (the party who institutes suit seeking relief) must prove certain components to prevail. If the jurisdiction adheres to the negligence theory of medical malpractice (which is the case in most states), these components are as follows:

1. The existence of the physician's duty to the plaintiff, usually based on the existence of the physician-patient relationship
2. The applicable standard of care and its violation
3. A compensable injury
4. A causal connection between the violation of the standard of care and the harm complained of[2]

One of the better-known minority theories of medical malpractice liability is referred to as the "Captain of the Ship" rule. This theory implements fundamental elements of what is known as the law of agency. Agency, simply stated, explains and defines the duties and obligations of those who act for and perform services for the benefit of others. Typically, an agency theory of law is incorporated into the Captain of the Ship rule in holding the physician liable for the acts of all—those parties assisting her or him before, during, and after surgery.

In most instances, even though those assisting parties are hospital employees, they are deemed to have been "temporary servants" of the physician while performing their services, and therefore the doctor becomes liable for their negligent acts.[3]

Certainly, the Captain of the Ship doctrine would afford the technologist a greater degree of insulation from medical malpractice liability. Unfortunately, this theory of law is diminishing under the weight of public opinion, which favors assessing liability on those who, by their acts or failure to act, have caused harm. Most jurisdictions adhere to the negligence theory of medical malpractice, in part because this theory seeks to hold all medical professionals accountable for their conduct. This appears to be the predominant view among the public as well.

In what is perceived by many to be an abusive tactic, many plaintiffs' lawyers in medical malpractice cases use what in the legal vernacular has been called the "buckshot" approach. This tactic implores the plaintiff to sue as many individuals and legal entities as came in contact with the plaintiff at or about the time when the injury was sustained. The objective is to "hit" (and presumably recover from) as many responsible parties as possible. These parties are not limited to physicians and nurses. Radiologic technologists are more likely to be named in suits along with multiple other defendants than they are to be the sole defendants.

In fairness to plaintiffs' counsel, the appellation of "buckshot" carries with it a pejorative taint. Most medical malpractice cases involve complex factual situations, serious injuries, and multiple care providers. Accordingly, they are likely to include multiple defendants.

How can radiologic technologists protect themselves from liability? The search for an answer to this question is consistent with containing medical malpractice costs and, consequently, would favorably affect health care costs in general.

It is my contention that clear definition is essential when dealing with the bounds of the technologist's role in the medical care arena. Definition will serve the profession well, while at the same time tend to narrow malpractice exposure and, hence, lower health care delivery costs.

Certainly, defining venipuncture and the administration of pharmacologic agents as within or outside the boundaries of the profession is important. Currently, the vast majority of states do not permit technologists to do so.

CURRENT PRACTICES AND THE LAW

In some states that prohibit technologist venipuncture by statute, there has been a widespread practice to work around this prohibition. This is particularly so in hospitals that rationalize that the procedure is being performed within the limits of the person's role as a hospital employee. This highly questionable (though widespread) practice is justified by "convenience" and "expedience." I interviewed a prominent Massachusetts radiologist who acknowledged that a technologist legally "can't give anything," but also acknowledged that venipuncture and contrast media administration does take place, hopefully at the direction of a physician. This same radiologist was aware that technologists did not receive training in pharmacology and learned the technique of venipuncture "on the job."

Although the administration of contrast agents has long been accepted practice, it is not without attendant risks. Though routinely performed thousands of times each week, negligence in this procedure has had catastrophic consequences, as Bettman has shown:

> The overall safety of contrast agents . . . is a difficult subject to address because of the wide range of adverse effects they can have, the various classification systems for side effects, and the many etiologic variables.[4]

In addition,

> . . . other complications ascribed to contrast agents [have] included alterations in myocardial function, alterations in renal function, vascular endothelial damage, and central nervous system depression.[4]

Inevitably, technologists have been named as defendants in lawsuits in which the plaintiff sustained severe injuries. These suits include an instance wherein the technologist was found liable after performing venipuncture that resulted in severe nerve damage to the patient.[5]

In another lawsuit, a technologist was sued for injuries sustained by a 23-month-old girl following an injection of a contrast medium into her calves, which allegedly caused the girl to suffer a shortening of the Achilles tendon, requiring surgery and the wearing of a corrective leg brace. The court indicated that technologists were not sufficiently trained in the administration of contrast media.[6]

When the technologist performs venipuncture and administers drugs, the level of exposure and potential liability inevitably rises. With this increase in actual and potential exposure comes the attendant insurance costs which, as was seen with doctors, negatively affect the financial aspects of practice. As doctors become more "insurance conscious," is it not good practice for the technologist to do so as well?

SUMMARY

The expansion of the practice of radiographic technology should be accomplished with the utmost of care. Technologists should not unwarily place themselves in the vacuum of malpractice liability left by doctors who have learned by experience. Technologists should learn from the physicians' experience in the field of malpractice and thereby limit their exposure. This is preferable to the hasty expansion of the profession into these two areas wherein national curricula, licensing, and statutory standards lag years behind.

Any technologist who now both performs venipuncture and administers drugs is subject to a reasonably high degree of risk, especially to malpractice actions. A serious or even unfavorable outcome to such a situation by a patient exposes the technologist to great peril. Accordingly, technologists who perform venipuncture in a state that prohibits them from doing so become ripe targets for plaintiffs' medical malpractice attorneys. In such jurisdictions, it is typically held that a "violation of statute" (the act of performing venipuncture by technologists) is evidence of negligence and therefore places the technologist in a vulnerable position. Furthermore, during the course of what is known as "discovery" (pretrial information gathering), a plaintiff's attorney could establish that the technologist had no or minimal training in pharmacology. The combination of statutory violation coupled with the lack of formal pharmacology training would all but assure a plaintiff's recovery against the technologist.

Although I am unwilling to take the position that the technologist should never administer drugs or perform venipuncture, now is decidedly not the time to do so. Certainly, there must first be a widespread revamping of current curricula throughout the country to include a detailed and comprehensive pharmacology component as well as clinical fieldwork in venipuncture. Certification standards would have to be expanded, after which there would be a legitimate need to amend the various state laws to permit these activities by technologists. Time constraints and the realities of politics make such a nationwide change unlikely in the near future. In the interim, in addition to new curricula, provisions would have to be made to retrain practicing technologists to meet new licensing and insurability standards.

Until the educational and legislative standards both are consistent and include venipuncture and drug administration, the profession should proceed with caution. When these standards become uniform nationwide, the technologist will be on much firmer ground to perform these services from both an education-competence perspective and a medicolegal malpractice perspective.

At that time, the profession will attain true legitimacy and public recognition as a competent vehicle for the delivery of these vital services. This is certainly preferable to the somewhat "off the record" methods now used in the many states in which venipuncture and pharmacological administration are not permitted by technologists.

In the interim, I would advise the profession to heed the Code of Ethics adopted by both the American Society of Radiologic Technologists and the American Registry of Radiologic Technologists, particularly paragraph 7: "The Radiologic Technologist utilizes equipment and accessories, employs techniques and procedures, performs services in accordance with an accepted standard of practice. . . ."[7]

I do not suggest that the profession remain stagnant. To the contrary, I agree with paragraph 10 of the Code of Ethics, which implores the technologist to "continually [strive] to improve knowledge and skills by participating in educational and professional activities, sharing knowledge with colleagues and investigating new and innovative aspects of professional practice. . . ."[7]

By so doing, public recognition will soon follow. With the requisite public recognition will come governmental regulation. When the various state regulating agencies become convinced that both the educational foundation and the public need exist, venipuncture and drug administration by technologists will become an accepted part of practice.

Until such time, prematurely embracing these techniques will ultimately prove to be counterproductive and actually lengthen the time before which these procedures will be legalized. Nothing positive will be accomplished by the technologist becoming a ripe target for malpractice and earning public enmity in the process.

By raising both educational goals and public awareness, the case for legalization will be strong. Until that time, the technologist would be well advised to practice within the legal limits of the profession. If the technologist wishes to effect a change, the way to do so is through legislative lobbying and not by performing impermissible procedures.

BIBLIOGRAPHY

1. O'Neil, EH: Health professions for the future: schools in service to the nation. Pew Health Professions Commission, San Francisco, 1993, p. 74.
2. Kosberg v. Washington Hospital Center, Inc., 129 U.S. App. D.C. 322, 394 F.2d 947, 949.
3. Ybarra v. Spangard, 25 Cal. 2d 486, 154 P.2d 687, 93 Cal. App. 2d 43, 208 P.2d 445.
4. Bettman, MA: Radiologic contrast agents—a perspective. N Engl J Med 317:892, October 1, 1987.
5. Montgomery v. Opelousas General Hospital, 540 So. 2d 312 (Ala. 1989).
6. Brook v. St. John's Hickeg Memorial Hospital, 368 N.E.2d 264 (Ind. 1977).
7. Code of Ethics, supra. Written by American Society of Radiologic Technologists and adopted by the American Registry of Radiologic Technologists. Albuquerque, July, 1994.

Pharmacology Overview

INTRODUCTION

Pharmacology is the science of the study of drugs and their uses, chemical composition, and interaction. To discuss all the aspects of pharmacology is beyond the scope of this text. However, a broad overview of pharmacology is necessary for persons administering drugs.

This chapter addresses the various divisions of pharmacology. These divisions are pharmacodynamics, pharmacokinetics, pharmacognosy, pharmacotherapeutics, and toxicology (Fig. 4–1). Pharmacodynamics deals with the biochemical effect, physical effect, and mechanism of action of a drug. Pharmacokinetics relates to the absorption, distribution, metabolism, and excretion of a drug. Determining the drug source is known as pharmacognosy. Pharmacotherapeutics concerns the clinical application of drugs. The study of the toxicity, harmful effects, and adverse reaction of drugs is known as toxicology.

Because of their importance, pharmacodynamics and pharmacokinetics will be discussed in detail. The remaining divisions will be briefly summarized. Prior to discussing these divisions, it is important to define the terms that are used in this chapter and that may appear in other chapters.

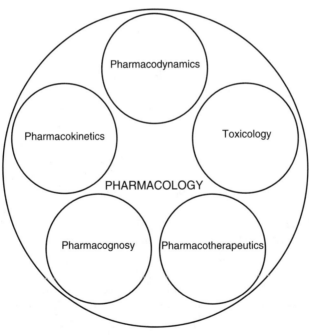

FIGURE 4–1
Pharmacology divisions.

NOMENCLATURE

The following definition of terms used throughout this text will help the reader to avoid semantic problems that may arise from different interpretations of words:

Adverse Reaction   An undesirable response to a drug by the patient. Adverse reactions are usually considered more severe than side effects.

Allergy   A response to a drug after a patient was previously exposed to the drug and developed antibodies to the drug.

Brand Name   See *Trade Name.*

Chemical Name   The drug's chemical (atomic and molecular) composition.

Dose   Amount of a drug needed to produce a specific effect.

Drug   A medication that can interact with a living organism to produce a biological effect. Drugs tend to be classified as *prescription* (used under supervision of a physician) and *nonprescription* (over the counter).

Drug Abuse   Excessive use of drugs for nontherapeutic reasons.

Drug Dependence   Psychological craving for or physiological reliance on a drug, often resulting from drug abuse or addiction.

Drug Efficacy   Maximum response or effect of a drug. It represents the peak of the drug-response curve.

Drug Misuse   Improper use of a drug that may cause acute and chronic toxicity.

Drug Potency   Amount of a drug needed to produce the desired response.

Generic Name   Name usually derived from the chemical name and the name manufacturers use. The name is assigned by the American Pharmaceutical Association, the American Medical Association, and the United States Adopted Names Council.

Iatrogenic Reaction   Occurs when a drug imitates or induces a disease.

Idiosyncratic Reaction   Any unusual or abnormal response to a drug.

Official Name   Name given by the Food and Drug Administration (FDA). A list of official drugs can be found in the United States Pharmacopeia (USP) and the National Formulary (NF).

Proprietary Name   See *Trade Name.*

Receptor Site   The specific location in a cell where the drug attaches and may or may not produce some type of cellular change.

Response   The effect of the drug.

Side Effect   Any reaction or adverse response to a drug.

Site of Action   Where the therapeutic effect of a drug occurs.

Trade Name   The name given to the drug by the manufacturer. The name is usually short, easy to remember, and descriptive of the drug. The trade name is protected by copyright.

DRUG SAFETY AND STANDARDS

The Food and Drug Administration (FDA) is the governmental agency that is responsible for ensuring that drugs used in the United States are safe. Companies interested in developing and marketing any new drug must perform several phases of drug testing.

The first step in the testing is animal testing. The tests are designed to obtain data regarding the safety and efficacy of the drug. The company submits the data to the FDA for their approval. If the drug is approved, the company may begin the Investigational New Drug (IND) testing phases.

In the IND testing, the drug first is given to a small number of healthy volunteers. If the human response to the drug is acceptable, the next step is to administer the medication to a small number of volunteers with the disease for which the drug is claimed to be effective. If testing of the small sample of "diseased" patients proves effective, the drug is administered to a much larger sample. After completing this process, the company provides the data from all phases of testing to the FDA and applies for a New Drug Application (NDA).

Upon FDA approval, the drug is made available to the public. However, the company must conduct a postmarket survey from physicians to determine the efficacy of the drug. During this time, the company must report the survey data to the FDA and the public. If the drug is found to be toxic, it is removed from the market.

This process often takes years before the drug receives approval. To date, the only drugs allowed to bypass the process or have the process expedited are the experimental drugs used in the treatment of acquired immunodeficiency syndrome (AIDS).

The United States publishes the Pharmacopeia of the United States of America (USP) and National Formulary (NF), which identify the standards for drugs used in the United States. These texts provide a great deal of information that includes, but is not limited to, the drug's purity, potency, dosage, and toxicity. Another publication is the USP Dispensing Information (DI), which contains information on dispensing and administering a drug.

The United Nations World Health Organization (WHO) attempts to provide international health care and information. One of the responsibilities of WHO is to establish drug standards, e.g., the standardization of drug names. This organization publishes Pharmacopoeia Internationalis (Ph. I.) in an effort to provide uniform drug standards. However, WHO has no legal or other means available to enforce its findings. Thus, the success of WHO largely depends on the cooperation of nations.

A common and popular reference used to locate information on drugs is the Physician's Desk Reference (PDR). This reference has several lists that can be used to find a specific drug. These include classification by product name, product category (clinical effect classification), generic and chemical name, and manufacturer's name. Of particular interest to technologists is the Diagnostic Product

Information section, which is an alphabetical listing, by manufacturer, of drugs used in diagnostic procedures. Besides the usual basic description of the drug, there are summaries of preprocedure care, considerations during the procedure, and postprocedural care.

DRUG CLASSIFICATIONS

Drugs may be classified in numerous ways. Some examples are classification by chemical composition, site of action, and route of administration. As such, it is possible for a specific drug to be located under several different classifications. The index categories used in the PDR are a typical example of the "multiple listings" of a drug relative to classification.

Two common classifications of drugs are by the clinical effect and by the effect on a specific body system. An example of drug classification by clinical effect is an antacid. A drug that would be listed under the antacid classification is sodium bicarbonate. The gastrointestinal system is an example of classification by specific body system. Sodium bicarbonate could also be listed in this area because it is a type of medication that is used for disorders of the gastrointestinal system.

PHARMACODYNAMICS

Pharmacodynamics is the study of the mechanisms by which drug dosages produce changes in the body. It is believed that the changes occur because of cellular or enzymatic interaction.

INTERACTION THEORIES

In the cellular interaction, a drug attaches itself to a receptor site (affinity) to initiate a biological change (efficacy). When a drug reaches its receptor site, it may produce different effects. For example, if the drug and receptor site "match" and a positive response occurs, the drug is referred to as an *agonist*. Drugs that have an affinity for a cell, but counteract or inhibit the action of other drugs, are called *antagonists*. There are two types of antagonist drugs: noncompetitive and competitive. *Noncompetitive antagonists* usually prevent, or "block," other drugs from producing an effect. Increasing the concentration of the agonist does not affect, or reverse, the antagonist's action. It is also possible for an antagonist drug to compete (called *competitive antagonism*) with an agonist drug. In these cases, it is possible to overcome the antagonist's effect by increasing the concentration of the agonists.

An enzymatic interaction is functionally comparable to what occurs according to the cellular receptor theory. However, instead of having an affinity for cells, the drug combines with an enzyme. The enzyme behaves as a cell receptor.

The number of receptors available is limited. When the drug has occupied all the receptors, an increase in dose does not increase the therapeutic effect.

DOSE-RESPONSE CURVE

It is possible to graph the relationship of the dose of a drug to its response or dose-response curve. These curves use the *effective dose 50* (ED 50), or dose needed to produce a response in 50% of the population, to compare the potency of different drugs producing the same response (Fig. 4–2). For example, in Figure 4–2, drug Y requires about 20 mg more to produce an effect similar to that of drug X (50 mg − 30 mg = 20 mg).

TIME-RESPONSE CURVE

When a drug is administered, there is a delay until it reaches its minimal effective concentration. After attaining the minimal effective concentration, the drug will produce a response for a specific time before its action or effectiveness becomes inactive (terminated). It is possible to demonstrate the onset of action, duration,

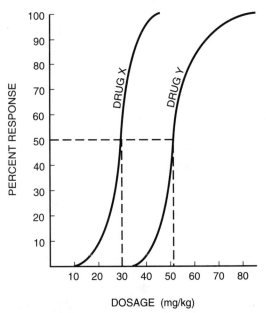

FIGURE 4–2
Dose-response curve for drugs X and Y.

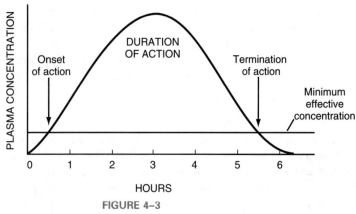

FIGURE 4–3
Time-response curve for drug X.

and termination rates by using a time-response graph (Fig. 4–3). These curves are useful in determining how frequently to administer a dose to maintain an effective drug response.

In Figure 4–3, the first effect (onset of action) is at 30 minutes. The length of time the drug is effective (duration of action) is 5 hours. After 5½ hours, the drug is no longer effective (termination of action). Thus, to maintain an effective response, one should administer the drug about every 5 hours.

THERAPEUTIC INDEX

The therapeutic index (TI) is a measure of degree of safety of a drug. The TI is determined by dividing the lethal dose 50 (LD 50) by the effective dose 50 (ED 50). This is written mathematically as: TI = LD 50 / ED 50. The LD 50 is the dosage of a drug that has been proven lethal in 50% of laboratory animals. ED 50 is the dose needed to produce a therapeutic effect in 50% of a population. The smaller the difference between LD 50 and ED 50 (or the closer the quotient is to 1), the smaller the safety margin. Patients who are given drugs with a small safety margin should be monitored closely.

FACTORS INFLUENCING DRUG RESPONSE

Many factors can affect the efficacy of a drug. The most common factors are body weight, age, emotional state, gender, genetics, and pathological status.

The weight of a person affects the amount of drug concentration and distribution in the body. Drug dosage is determined when it is effective in 50% of the population weighing about 150 pounds (70 kg) and between the ages of 18 and 65. Dose adjustments need to be made for individuals who are ±50 pounds (100 and 200 pounds). An increased dose is needed for larger patients, whereas a decreased dose is required for smaller patients. The amount to increase or decrease is determined by the physician. Often the pamphlet insert that comes with the drug includes a suggested dose by patient weight, age, or both.

As previously mentioned, dosage is determined for an age range of 18 to 65 years. Infants, children, and the elderly require a different dose. Doses for such persons tend to be smaller than the average adult dose. In infants and children, the dose is reduced because of immature enzymatic, renal, and hepatic systems. The elderly require a smaller dose because of possible reduced functions of the hepatic, renal, or other systems.

The psychological belief of the individual in medicine and drugs has an extremely strong effect on the drug's efficacy. The strongest evidence of how an individual's psychological drug expectation influences response is the placebo effect. Patients who have great faith in drugs and medicine have been given inert drugs instead of an actual medication and have had their condition improve. Conversely, individuals who tend to be hostile or negative to drugs have showed no improvement when administered a drug.

There is some controversy as to the effect of gender on drug response. In general, it is believed that because women have more body fat and tend to be smaller than men that a smaller dose should be given to women. Also, because drugs are known to affect the fetus, the type and amount of drug given to pregnant women should be limited.

Individuals tend to inherit the traits of their parents. This may include the parent's ability to respond to drugs. If a parent has problems with drug response, it is possible that the child will inherit the same difficulties.

Some diseases may adversely affect the patient's response to a drug. Because most drugs are metabolized by the liver and excreted through the kidneys, any deficiency in the renal or hepatic systems tends to increase the possibility of an adverse reaction or alter the effectiveness of a drug.

ADVERSE REACTIONS

Sometimes drugs produce an unwanted effect. An undesirable response to a drug is known as an *adverse reaction*. The term adverse reaction tends to be reserved for responses that are more severe than a side effect, which is a mild and tolerable reaction to a drug. There are several types of adverse reactions. These include allergic, idiosyncratic, and iatrogenic.

An allergy is a response to a drug that occurs when a patient was previously exposed to the drug and developed antibodies to the drug. When the body is re-exposed to the drug to which the person is allergic, an antigen-antibody reaction occurs, producing an adverse effect on other parts of the body. An allergic reaction may be mild, e.g., rash, or more serious, or even fatal. The reaction may occur immediately or be delayed, e.g., occurring several days after drug administration.

Immediate and severe reactions are called *anaphylactic*. Persons with known allergies should avoid use of the drug to which they are allergic.

An idiosyncratic reaction is any unusual or abnormal response to a drug. This term is often used to refer to reactions other than allergic responses. Idiosyncratic reactions are thought to occur because of genetic or hormonal enzymatic deficiencies.

Iatrogenic reactions are those in which the drug imitates or induces a disease. Common syndromes seen in iatrogenic reactions are blood dyscrasia, hepatic toxicity, renal injury, malformations of the fetus, and dermatological effects.

PHARMACOKINETICS

The pharmacodynamic phase occurs simultaneously with the pharmacokinetic stage. Pharmacokinetics is the science dealing with the absorption, distribution, metabolism, and excretion of a drug from a living organism.

ABSORPTION

Absorption is the process by which a drug is assimilated in the body after its administration. The rate and amount of absorption of a drug depends on the route of administration, drug solubility, and the blood flow to the site.

Route of Administration

The number of classifications of drug administration varies according to what text is used to define the categories. In this text, four primary means of drug administration are identified. They are enteral, parenteral, pulmonary, and topical. Some texts list two classifications, parenteral and enteral, whereas others add a third, topical.

In the enteral method, the absorption of the drug occurs in the gastrointestinal (GI) tract. In this method, drugs are available in a variety of forms, which include pills (tablets and capsules), liquids, suppositories, and granules. Administration of these drugs is by sublingual (under the tongue), buccal (drug is placed between the gum and cheek), oral, or rectal means.

Because of the potential for consumer product tampering, nonprescription products have a protective seal. A broken seal indicates that the product may have been tampered with and the drug should not be used.

This text defines the parenteral route as administration by injection. This includes intravenous, intra-arterial, intramuscular, intradermal, intrathecal, and subcutaneous injections. Most parenteral drugs are in liquid form and tend to be administered by medical personnel.

Pulmonary administration uses inhalation to direct the drug to the lungs. The medication may be in the form of fine mists or gases.

The topical route employs the application of a cream, liquid, or ointment to a specific part of the body. The most common areas requiring topical administration are the skin, eyes, and ears.

Enteral Administration

Of the enteral methods, the oral approach is the most common. In general, the average absorption rate for oral administration is 30–60 minutes, whereas the rectal method has an absorption rate of about 15–30 minutes. Sublingual and buccal administrations are the fastest enteral methods, with absorption occurring within minutes. Although the absorption may occur in different parts of the GI tract, e.g., gastric mucosa, absorption primarily occurs in the small intestine with the oral method. Absorption in the GI tract usually results in the medication being filtered through the liver before entering the blood stream. Sublingual, buccal, and rectal drugs bypass the liver and enter the blood stream directly through membrane absorption. The design of oral medications determines the absorption location and rate. For example, some pills are coated to prevent gastric secretions from acting on the drug. Some granules have different thicknesses of protective coating that permit dissolution at different rates ("time released"). As with all medications, the patient should be provided proper instructions for their administration. Some common precautions that should be adhered to for oral medications are:

- Never chew medications unless instructed to do so.
- Unscored tablets (pills without the appropriate "impression" or line used to divide the dose) should not be cut.
- Follow the proper instructions for taking medications, e.g., take with water, don't take with food, etc.
- Do not open capsules containing granules.
- When using sublingual drugs, refrain from swallowing saliva as long as possible.

Parenteral Administration

Although less common than the enteral method, parenteral administration of drugs is preferred when a more rapid drug response is needed. In general, the type of parenteral administration determines the speed of drug response. The slowest absorption rate, taking hours, occurs with the intradermal (e.g., allergy testing) method. The subcutaneous, intramuscular, and intrathecal methods take several minutes before a drug response is observed. Intravenous and intra-arterial methods yield an extremely rapid response, within a minute.

Pulmonary Administration

The use of inhalers for drug administration results in rapid absorption of the drug. Many of these drugs are designed to produce a rapid local effect and are readily absorbed in the alveolar sacs.

Topical Administration

The three areas most often targeted for topical drugs are the skin, eyes, and ears. Most topical drugs are designed to produce a local response. When applying a topical solution to the skin, one should administer it to an area that has no openings (cuts). A topical solution that enters the blood stream though a cut could result in an adverse reaction.

Transdermal patches are another form of topical administration of drugs. In this method, a patch containing medication is applied to the intact, unshaven skin. The patches allow a continuous delivery of the drug. Certain drug patches may be worn for up to 1 week or longer before applying a new one. The location of the patch should be rotated to different body parts to avoid skin irritation. Also, the location of the patch should be in accordance with the manufacturer's recommendation. Some patches may need to be applied to the chest, whereas others are applied to the extremities.

Drug Solubility

Solubility is the ability of a drug to dissolve. The rate at which the drug dissolves is influenced by the form of medication—that is, the cellular composition must match the drug. For example, lipid medications can penetrate lipid cells, whereas water soluble drugs cannot. Other factors that can affect the solubility include coating pills so that they absorb slowly, taking medications with water to increase solubility, and using oily drugs for injection to slow absorption.

Blood Flow

In general, the greater the blood flow to the absorption site, the faster the absorption. A variety of factors affect the flow of blood. Food tends to stimulate blood flow, increasing absorption. An intramuscular injection in the deltoid muscle results in faster absorption of the drug, but a larger dose can be given if administered in the gluteal muscle. Blood flow can be increased by massaging or applying heat to the injection site. A decrease in blood flow can be obtained by cooling the injection site or applying a tourniquet proximal to the point of administration.

DISTRIBUTION

Once a drug is absorbed by the body, it is dispersed throughout the body and to the site of action via the blood circulation and lymphatic systems. This process is known as distribution. During distribution, the drug accumulates, or is stored, in various parts of the body. This accumulation is responsible for "prolonging" the effect of the drug. Three factors affect the accumulation of the drug. They are plasma protein binding, blood flow, and blood barriers.

Drugs are either free or bind with plasma protein (drug protein complex). Free drugs are active and able to produce a pharmacological effect. Drugs attached to plasma protein are inactive and do not produce a response. However, the ratio of free drugs to bound drug complexes in circulation is constant. This means that as the free drug is excreted, the drug protein complexes begin to disassociate, or "detach," from the protein plasma to become free drug molecules. Plasma protein binding is expressed as a percentage. For example, 90% of the molecules may be bound in a highly protein-binding drug. This means that 10% are free and active. A decrease in the percentage of plasma proteins limits the amount of storage and increases the amount of free drug in the blood. Malnutrition, renal disease, and liver disease tend to decrease the level of plasma proteins. In these cases, the dosage should be adjusted appropriately. Care should be taken when patients are taking multiple drugs. Drugs with a high protein-binding percentage may compete with other drugs for the binding sites and displace them.

The greater the amount of blood flow to an organ, the more exposure that organ has to the drug. Organs with large blood flows include the heart, liver, kidney, and brain. These organs tend to receive the majority of the initial drug administered. The muscles and fat have a relatively low blood supply and don't tend to accumulate much of the drug.

The body has two natural barriers to drug absorption. They are the blood-brain barrier and the placental barrier. The blood-brain barrier occurs because the cells in the brain allow only lipid-soluble compounds. Because most drugs are not fat soluble, they don't enter the brain. However, it is possible to bypass the blood circulation of the brain by administering drugs intrathecally. The membranes and enzymes of the placenta act as a barrier to the intrusion of some drugs. However, many drugs can penetrate the placenta and enter the fetus.

METABOLISM

The body tends to rid itself of foreign substances such as drugs. Some drugs are eliminated from the body in their original form, whereas others must undergo a chemical change. The objective is to transform a drug, usually lipid soluble, from its original state to a water-soluble state for excretion. The process of the body altering the chemical composition of material is called *metabolism*. The result of metabolism is a metabolite. In the case of medications, the metabolite is often in the form of an inactive drug. Most chemical changes occur by enzymatic action of the liver. This is commonly referred to as the drug microsomal metabolizing system, or DMMS. Some drugs stimulate metabolic activity and become more active, creating serious adverse reactions. Certain diseases also affect metabolism. Persons with liver disease, congestive heart failure, or severe renal dysfunction tend to have a lengthened metabolism rate. Genetic make-up may also alter the rate of metabolism. Infants and the aged tend to have a prolonged metabolism rate.

EXCRETION

The process of eliminating wastes or unwanted material from the body is called *excretion*. The body may eliminate these materials in a variety of ways. Common forms of excretion include elimination via the GI tract, kidneys, and lungs. Less common routes for eliminating byproducts are the exocrine glands (skin, salivary glands, and mammary glands). The length of time it takes for metabolism and excretion varies. A common method to represent this time is the half-life of the drug. Half-life is the time required by the body to eliminate 50% of the drug. Most drugs are essentially eliminated after 5 half-lives. Half-life is also useful in determining the duration of action of the drug, which is valuable when determining the time between doses.

PHARMACOGNOSY

Pharmacognosy deals with the sources of drugs. There are four main sources of drugs. They are plants, animals, minerals or mineral products, and synthetic chemical substances. Original drugs were obtained from natural sources, e.g., plants, and consisted of a "dry" or powder form. In the early development of drugs, many medications contained inert or multiple active ingredients. As time progressed, the process of making drugs became more sophisticated, resulting in "pure" medications. Modern medical advances now allow the profession to synthesize drugs. However, there are no true 100% synthetic drugs. Most medications are an alteration of a natural substance.

Drugs contain active ingredients and additives. The active ingredient is responsible for the action of the drug. Most prescription drugs contain one active ingredient, whereas "over the counter" medications tend to have multiple active ingredients. Additives are substances attached to the drug to produce a specific function or property to the drug. There are several types of additives. Common examples of substances added are flavor, a filler to provide a uniform dose, a vehicle (e.g., water, oils) to provide the shape and substance of drug, material to improve the cohesiveness of dry drugs (binders), and materials to improve the appearance (dyes). Additives should be compatible with the active ingredient and not interact with it or change it.

PHARMACOTHERAPEUTICS

Pharmacotherapeutics is a science that includes drugs used for the diagnosis, prevention, and treatment of disease. Many diagnostic drugs are used in radiology, e.g., contrast media. Preventive medications are used to avert diseases. Vaccinations are typical preventive medications.

There are a variety of ways to treat disease. Much of the decision as to which method to use depends on the type and stage of the disease. Common therapies are supportive, palliative, maintenance, and supplemental or replacement. Supportive therapy occurs when a patient is administered a drug to prevent the disease from injuring other organs or body systems. This type of treatment is common in viral infections. Patients receiving palliative therapy are usually in the latter stages of a terminal disease. Often, the drugs administered are the type used to relieve pain. Maintenance therapy is used in chronically ill patients whose disease continues, e.g., hypertension. This therapy is used to prevent damage and maintain a normal health level. Supplemental or replacement therapy is used to add or replace substances the body does not have or produce, e.g., insulin.

It is important in pharmacotherapeutics to determine the correct dose and monitor the effects of the medication. Numerous factors affect dose (see "Pharmacodynamics" and "Pharmacokinetics"). Sometimes multiple drugs are used in therapy to obtain a synergistic (greater) effect.

TOXICOLOGY

The science of toxicology is broad and includes analysis of other than medicinal drugs, e.g., environmental toxicology. The treatment for adverse reaction to drugs varies. A basic step to treat poisoning is to eliminate the source. This may be done by emesis, lavage (pumping the stomach), or cathartics. The most commonly known treatment is to provide an antidote. An antidote is designed to counteract the toxic material.

Most major cities have a poison center. A list of poison center locations can be obtained by writing the FDA's National Clearinghouse for Poison Control Centers in Bethesda, MD. The front of local telephone books generally lists the number of the closest center.

BIBLIOGRAPHY

Bentley, PJ: Elements of pharmacology, a primer on drug action. Cambridge University Press, New York, 1981.

Edmunds, MW: Introduction to clinical pharmacology. Mosby Yearbook, St. Louis, 1991.

Ehrlich, RA and McCloskey, ED: Patient care in radiography. Mosby Yearbook, St. Louis, 1993.

Hahn, AB, Oestreich, SJK, Barkin, RL, et al: Mosby's Pharmacology in Nursing. CV Mosby, St. Louis, 1986.

Hitner, H, and Nagle, BT: Basic pharmacology for health occupations. Bobbs-Merrill Educational Publishing, Indianapolis, 1980.

Schwertz, DW: Basic principles of pharmacologic action. Nurs Clin North Am 26(2):2, 1991.

Spencer, RT, Nichols, LW, Lipkin, GB, et al: Clinical pharmacology and nursing management, 3rd edition. JB Lippincott, Philadelphia, 1989.

Torres, LS: Basic medical techniques and patient care for radiologic technologists, 4th edition. JB Lippincott, Philadelphia, 1993.

Williams, BR, and Baer, CL: Essentials of clinical pharmacology in nursing. Springhouse Corporation, Springhouse, PA, 1990.

Drug Measurements and Dose Calculation

5

INTRODUCTION

Drugs may only be administered with a prescription from an appropriate licensed person, e.g., a physician. Once a prescription is written, the appropriate dose (quantity) is prepared for administration. Three systems are used to measure the dose: the metric, apothecary, and household systems. The manner in which the drug is supplied and the method the physician uses to order the drug dictate the system used for the dose. Sometimes the physician orders the drug using one system, but the drug is supplied using a different system. Consequently, it is important to understand how to convert from one system to another.

This chapter discusses prescriptions, types of systems used to measure dose, the conversion of dose between and within systems, and computing dosage.

PRESCRIPTIONS

States regulate the licensing of physicians. One of the privileges of a licensed physician is the right to prescribe drugs. Some states have extended that right to physician assistants, nurse practitioners, and other health care workers. However, these people often have "limited" prescription writing powers, e.g., they are unable to order controlled substances. Also, many states require that the orders be written under the direct supervision of a physician.

Persons writing prescriptions should include the name, address, and age of the patient; the date; the medication name; the dose and interval of doses (frequency); the route of administration; and the signature of the person licensed to prescribe the drug on the prescription. It is common for the information on a prescription to contain abbreviations. The abbreviations usually have a Greek or Latin origin. Table 5–1 lists common abbreviations used or apt to be seen in an imaging department. Additional information that may be included on prescriptions includes whether or not the person dispensing the drug can use a generic substitute and the number of refills. Prescriptions may be written or verbal (via telephone).

Written prescriptions contain the information just described and are recorded on paper. The written prescription is given to the person preparing the drug for dispensing. Verbal orders are usually received by telephone. The person receiving the order records all the necessary information on a prescription form. The name of the person ordering the drug and initials of the person taking the order are also recorded on the prescription. The person ordering the medication must sign the prescription as soon as the person is available to do so.

SYSTEM OF MEASURES AND WEIGHTS

The dosage ordered is written in one of the three measurement systems. The systems are metric, apothecary, and household. These systems vary significantly.

TABLE 5–1

Common Abbreviations Used on Prescriptions

Abbreviation	Meaning
Frequency of Dose	
ad lib	as desired
b.i.d.	twice a day
p.c.	after meals
PRN	as required
t.i.d.	3 times a day
q.d.	every day
q.i.d.	four times a day
Quantity of Dose	
cc	cubic centimeter
fl oz	fluid ounce
g	gram
L	liter
ml	milliliter
T or Tbs	tablespoon
t or tsp	teaspoon
Method of Administration	
IM	intramuscular
IV	intravenous
PO	oral
SC	subcutaneous
SL	sublingual

It is difficult to move from one system to another and maintain the exact quantity. Most conversions are close approximates. The following is a brief summary of each system.

METRIC SYSTEM

The metric system was developed in France in the late 1700s to standardize weights and measures. It is the most popular system and is used by most nations of the world. In this system, the unit of length is the meter. The liter is the unit for volume and the gram is the unit employed for weight.

The uniqueness of the metric system is that fractions of units are in multiples or divisions of 10 (Table 5–2). A unit fraction is identified by placing a prefix before the unit. The prefix determines whether the quantity is divided or a multiple of 10. The prefixes deci (0.1), centi (0.01), milli (0.001), and micro (0.000001)

TABLE 5–2

Metric Equivalents

Subdivision Unit	Basic Unit Equivalent
Length (Basic unit = meter)	
1 decimeter	0.1 meter
1 centimeter	0.01 meter
1 millimeter	0.001 meter
1 micrometer	0.000001 meter
1 decameter	10 meters
1 hectometer	100 meters
1 kilometer	1000 meters
Volume (Basic unit = liter)	
1 deciliter	0.1 liter
1 centiliter	0.01 liter
1 milliliter	0.001 liter
1 microliter	0.000001 liter
1 decaliter	10 liters
1 hectoliter	100 liters
1 kiloliter	1000 liters
Weight (Basic unit = gram)	
1 decigram	0.1 gram
1 centigram	0.01 gram
1 milligram	0.001 gram
1 microgram	0.000001 gram
1 decagram	10 grams
1 hectogram	100 grams
1 kilogram	1000 grams

represent the need to divide. For example, a centimeter is 0.01 or 1/100th of a meter. The prefixes deca (10), hecto (100), and kilo (1000) represent the need to multiply. For example, a kilometer is 1000 meters. It should be noted that these prefixes are also used with the gram and liter units.

The metric system was originally designed to permit easy transfer from one unit of measure to another. For example, one equivalency of volume to length is the liter (volume) and cubic decimeter (length), which are designed to be equal. In reality, the liter is slightly larger than a cubic decimeter by 28 parts per million. However, the difference is so small that in practice they are considered equal. Also, the derivatives of the liter and decimeter commonly used for dose (the milliliter, ml, and cubic centimeter, cc) are considered equal. The equivalency of weight to volume is 1 liter of water at 4° centigrade and weighs 1 kilogram (1000 grams).

APOTHECARY SYSTEM

The apothecary system is more cumbersome and less precise than the metric system. The United States is one of the few countries that still uses this system. However, the majority of measurements and weights used in the medical area in the United States are based on the metric system. Few medical areas employ the apothecary system.

The apothecary system consists of measures for liquids and solids. The minim is the basic unit for fluid volume and the grain is the unit employed for solids. Other units derived from the minim are the fluid ounce, pint, quart, and gallon. Units derived from the grain include the dram, ounce, and pound. Table 5–3 is a summary of the respective derivatives. It can be noted from Table 5–3 that, unlike the metric system, the divisions of the basic units in apothecary are cumbersome and are not multiples or divisions of 10.

HOUSEHOLD SYSTEM

The household system is the least desirable of the three systems used to measure dose. The system uses measures that are commonly found in a household. As the health care system relies more on home care, the household system becomes increasingly important. However, these measures are so crude that they should be avoided when precise quantities are necessary.

The measures used in the household system are most similar to the apothecary system. Unfortunately, there is little or no standardization of the measures. The most common dose units in household measures are the teaspoon, tablespoon, cup, and glass. It is possible to convert metric measurements to the apothecary system. For example, 1 teaspoon in the apothecary system equals 5 cc in the

TABLE 5–3

Apothecaries' Derivatives

Derivative	Equivalent
Liquid Measures (minim = basic unit)	
fluid dram	60 minims
fluid ounce	8 fluid drams
pint	16 fluid ounces
quart	2 pints
gallon	4 quarts
Solid Measures (grain = basic unit)	
dram	60 grains
ounce	8 drams
pound	12 ounces

metric system. Thus, if over-the-counter drug instructions require a dose of 10 cc, the person could use 2 teaspoons (10/5 = 2).

CONVERSIONS

The dose ordered and the dose administered must be in the same unit. As mentioned previously, measures must sometimes be converted. The primary types of conversions are within a system and between systems. The actual number of different conversions that may occur are numerous and beyond the scope of this text. Examples will be limited to those most commonly found in imaging departments. Table 5–4 compares the approximate equivalent measures of the three systems.

WITHIN A SYSTEM

Of the three systems, the metric system is the easiest for conversion from one unit to another. Conversion occurs by either multiplying or dividing by 10. The "shortcut" method is to move the decimal point to the right one "space" for every increment of 10. For example, 1.0 kilometer is equivalent to 1000.0 meters (the decimal is moved three spaces to the right). When the need exists to divide by 10, the decimal point is moved to the left one space for every increment of 1/10. For example, 1 milliliter is equivalent to 0.001 liters (the decimal is moved three spaces to the left). The key to determine whether the decimal moves to the right or to the left is the prefix. The decimal is moved to the left for prefixes requiring division and to the right for those that are multiples of 10.

The apothecary and household systems are more difficult to convert. To calculate the unknown factor, a proportion of the unit equivalent, the amount on hand, and desired amount is established. For example, determine how many drams are in 6 fluid ounces. The proportion of unit equivalent is 1 fluid ounce

TABLE 5–4

Metric, Apothecary, and Household Equivalents

Metric	Apothecary	Household
4–5 ml	1 dram	1 teaspoon
15 ml	4 drams	1 tablespoon
180 ml	6 oz	1 cup
240 ml	8 oz	1 glass

equals 8 fluid drams. The amount on hand is 6 fluid ounces and the unknown is "X" drams. Mathematically, this is written:

$$\frac{1 \text{ fluid ounce}}{8 \text{ fluid drams}} = \frac{6 \text{ fluid ounces}}{X}$$
$$(1)\ X = (6)\ (8)$$
$$X = 48 \text{ drams}$$

If the problem was reversed, or the question was how many fluid ounces are in 48 drams, the calculation is:

$$\frac{1 \text{ fluid ounce}}{8 \text{ fluid drams}} = \frac{X}{48 \text{ drams}}$$
$$(8)\ X = (1)\ (48)$$
$$8X = 48$$
$$X = 6 \text{ fluid ounces}$$

The proportion of unit equivalent is 1 fluid ounce equals 8 fluid drams. The amount on hand is 48 drams and the unknown is "X" fluid ounces. Notice, in both examples, that the numerators and denominators consist of the same unit, i.e., fluid ounces or drams.

BETWEEN SYSTEMS

The easiest way to convert a unit from one system to another is to look up the equivalent quantity on a chart (see Table 5–4). If the exact equivalent is not listed, to obtain the correct answer, set up a ratio so that each side (left and right) contains the same system unit. The numerators should be the equivalents in each system, e.g., 5 ml = 1 teaspoon. Sometimes it may be necessary to first change the unit within the system before converting it to another system. For example, if the chart uses liters and the problem is asking for milliliters, the liters must first be changed to milliliters. The denominator should be in the same system as the numerator above it; e.g., if the numerator is in milliliters, the denominator below it is also in milliliters. The following are examples of conversion between systems.

PROBLEM: How many milliliters are in 4 ounces?

$$240 \text{ ml} = 8 \text{ oz}$$
$$\frac{240 \text{ ml}}{X \text{ ml}} = \frac{8 \text{ oz}}{4 \text{ oz}}$$
$$8X = 960$$
$$X = 120 \text{ ml}$$

PROBLEM: How many ounces are in 500 cc?

$$1 \text{ cc} = 1 \text{ ml}$$
$$240 \text{ ml} = 8 \text{ oz}$$
$$240 \text{ cc} = 8 \text{ oz}$$
$$\frac{240 \text{ cc}}{500 \text{ cc}} = \frac{8 \text{ oz}}{X \text{ oz}}$$
$$240X = 4000$$
$$X = 16.6 \text{ oz}$$

COMPUTING DOSAGE

It is important that the units ordered, those available, and the unit administered be in the same system. Therefore, prior to calculating dosage, it is important to determine if the units must first be converted (see above).

After the units are converted, a simple formula is used to calculate the correct dose. It is:

$$\frac{\text{Dose ordered}}{\text{Dose available}} = \frac{\text{quantity administered}}{\text{volume available}}$$

The dose ordered is the amount of the drug the physician prescribes. The dose available represents how the drug unit is supplied, e.g., milligrams. Volume available refers to the volume of the drug that contains the dose available, e.g., tablet, milliliters. The quantity administered is the actual amount of the drug given to the patient. Often times the amount ordered, the dose available, and the volume available are in values that are easily calculated and do not require the use of the formula. For example, if a doctor orders 50 mg of a medication to be given to the patient and the drug available is 50 mg in a volume of 1 tablet, the quantity administered is 1 tablet. Mathematically, this would be:

$$\frac{50 \text{ mg}}{50 \text{ mg}} = \frac{X \text{ tablets}}{1 \text{ tablet}}$$
$$50X = 50$$
$$X = 1 \text{ tablet}$$

Besides performing the mathematics, it is important to use common sense. For example, suppose a physician orders 250 mg of a medication and the medication dose available is 125 mg per volume of 1 ml. Just by looking at the data provided, the dose required is greater than the amount available. Consequently, the volume administered should be greater than 1 ml. The correct calculation is:

$$\frac{250 \text{ mg}}{125 \text{ mg}} = \frac{X \text{ ml}}{1 \text{ ml}}$$
$$125X = 250$$
$$X = 2 \text{ ml}$$

If the contents in milligrams are accidentally transposed, the result is:

$$\frac{125 \text{ mg}}{250 \text{ mg}} = \frac{X \text{ ml}}{1 \text{ ml}}$$
$$250X = 125$$
$$X = 0.5 \text{ ml}$$

Visual observation of the answer, 0.5 ml, should alert the user that something is wrong because the administered dose is less than 1 ml.

Sometimes the calculation results in a fraction of a dose. This is especially true when determining the amount of "dry" oral medication, e.g., tablets or capsules, to administer. Sometimes dry medications, e.g., tablets, are "scored" (a "line" divides the tablet), allowing them to be broken so that smaller doses can be given. If the dry medication is not scored and the calculated dose results in the need to administer a fraction of the dose available, then when the quantity required is greater than 0.5, administer another dose available, e.g., a tablet. For example, if the calculated administered dose is 2.66 tablets, 3 tablets should be administered. For values less than 0.5, administer a lesser dose. For example, if the calculated administered dose is 2.32 tablets, 2 tablets should be administered.

Some medications are infused into the body using an intravenous (IV) "drip" method. Usually the drug mixture is prepared commercially by a nurse or pharmacist. The dose administered is determined by the flow rate of the solution.

The flow rate is measured by the number of drops per minute or "drop factor." The number of drops per minute varies with the equipment used and is located on the packaging of the equipment. Most infusion sets deliver 10–15 drops per minute. To determine the dosage (flow rate or drops per minute), the drop factor is multiplied by the volume to be delivered per minute. For example, if the drug is to be delivered at a volume of 3 ml/min and the drop factor is 10, the number of drops per minute is 30, or:

$$10 \times 3 \text{ ml/min} = 30$$

Two methods are used to regulate the flow rate. One is by manually adjusting the "roller clamp" located on the IV tubing. The other is by using an automatic infusion pump (Fig. 5–1). The infusion pumps have a more accurate rate of delivery than manual regulation of the infusion tubing. The pumps can regulate flow by counting the drops per minute or measuring the volume per minute. Because drop size may vary with the type of solution, the measurement in volume per minute is more accurate.

Sometimes the technologist must administer or assist in the administration of contrast medium to children. The amount of contrast medium administered to a child is based on the weight of the child. The recommended quantity to use per patient's weight is located in the contrast medium's package insert. The quantity is usually provided in cubic centimeters or milliliters and the weight is in kilograms (kg). Because the United States unit for weight is the pound (lb),

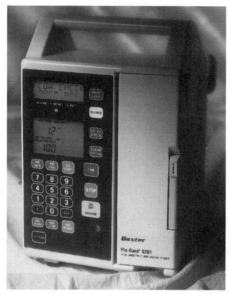

FIGURE 5–1
A Baxter Flo Gard 6201 infusion pump.

the technologist must convert the child's weight from pounds to kilograms. This is easily performed by dividing the weight of the patient by the number of pounds that equal 1 kg, or 2.2. For example, if the child weighs 66 lb, the weight in kilograms is 30, or 66/2.2 = 30. If the contrast medium insert suggests the administration of 0.5 ml/kg, the 66-lb child would receive 15 ml of contrast medium, or 0.5 × 30 = 15.

Certain contrast medium is manufactured as a powder and sealed in a glass vial. The manufacturer commonly produces contrast medium vials of different concentrations. The packaging of this type of contrast medium contains an aqueous diluent and the vial containing the contrast medium. To use the contrast medium, the diluent must be mixed with the contrast medium. The quantity of diluent and contrast medium used depends on the number of milligrams of iodine per milliliter (mgI/ml) desired. The package insert contains a chart of the recommended dosage for the examination and a table that identifies the amount of diluent to mix with the various contrast medium concentrations. For example, the dosage chart of Amipaque suggests a mgI/ml of 220 for thoracic myelography. To obtain the 220 mgI/ml, the technologist locates 220 mgI/ml on the diluent table. To determine the amount of milliliters of diluent, the technologist matches the 220 mgI/ml with the correct contrast medium concentration column, e.g., 6.75 g. This is achieved by "moving" along the 220 mgI/ml row until reaching the 6.75 g column. In this example, 11.7 ml of diluent is recommended. Because it is rather difficult to withdraw 11.7 ml, it is acceptable to use the closest ml value of 12 ml. The package insert identifies the maximum number of milliliters that could be safely employed.

BIBLIOGRAPHY

Chesney, DN, and Chesney, MO: Care of the patient in diagnostic radiography, 6th edition. Blackwell Scientific Publications, Boston, 1986.

Edmunds, MW: Introduction to clinical pharmacology. Mosby Yearbook, St. Louis, 1991.

Hahn, AB, Oestreich, SJK, Barkin, RL, et al: Mosby's pharmacology in nursing. CV Mosby, St. Louis, 1986.

Scherer, JC: Introductory clinical pharmacology, 3rd edition. JB Lippincott, Philadelphia, 1987.

Spencer, RT, et al: Clinical pharmacology and nursing management, 3rd edition. JB Lippincott, Philadelphia, 1989.

Contrast Media

JOSEPH R. BITTENGLE, M.Ed., ARRT(R)

DONNA C. DAVIS, M.Ed., ARRT(R)(CV)

6

INTRODUCTION

Because the x-ray absorption characteristics of structures such as the abdominal aorta and kidneys are nearly identical to those of the surrounding tissue structures, it is difficult to identify them on a routine anteroposterior abdominal projection. The gray densities of the abdominal contents tend to blend together, making visualization of discrete anatomical details nearly impossible.

The introduction of a radiopaque radiographic contrast medium into a structure such as the abdominal aorta or renal artery increases that tissue's ability to absorb x-ray photons. The anatomical structure filled with contrast medium produces a lighter, whiter image relative to the surrounding darker or grayer abdominal images. Thus, the edges of the contrast medium–filled areas are clearly outlined, and anatomical details are sharper and more apparent than on the radiograph taken without contrast medium.

Many specialized radiological examinations require the administration of a contrast medium during the procedure. The parenteral administration of a contrast medium, the various types of contrast media and their specific properties, some examples of the use of contrast media in clinical practice, and some precautions in the use of contrast media are discussed in this chapter.

PARENTERAL INJECTION METHODS

Parenteral drug administration methods include all means of administering a medication that bypass the patient's digestive system. Examples of parenteral drug administration methods include the topical route and intradermal, intramuscular, subcutaneous, intravenous, intra-arterial, and intrathecal injections. The three injection routes discussed in this chapter—intravenous, intra-arterial, and intrathecal—account for the majority of the types of contrast medium administration methods utilized during radiological procedures.

INTRAVENOUS

With the intravenous method, the contrast medium is infused or injected directly into the patient's venous circulatory system. A slow infusion of the contrast medium may be made into an easily accessible vein through a direct venipuncture using a venous catheter or angiocatheter. An example of a radiological examination that uses an infusion method for delivering the contrast medium is drip infusion pyelography (DIP), which is still performed in some facilities to demonstrate the urinary system. A bolus injection of the contrast medium may be made directly into the vein or via a *piggyback* method into a pre-existing venous line. An example of a radiological examination that uses a bolus injection of the contrast medium is intravenous pyelography (IVP), which is a more common radiographic procedure to demonstrate the urinary system. Whether an infusion or an injection method is chosen, both require the use of strict aseptic technique.

INTRA-ARTERIAL

The intra-arterial method of administering an iodinated contrast medium entails the injection of the contrast medium directly into the patient's arterial circulatory system. Following the selective catheterization of an arterial vessel, iodinated contrast medium is injected through the catheter into the desired arterial vessel. An example of a radiological examination that uses an intra-arterial injection of the iodinated contrast medium is the coronary angiogram performed during a cardiac catheterization procedure to demonstrate the coronary arteries. The use of strict surgical asepsis is mandatory.

INTRATHECAL

The intrathecal, or intraspinal, method of administering an iodinated contrast medium is the injection of the contrast medium through a spinal needle directly into the patient's meningeal subarachnoid space. Common intrathecal administration methods include the lumbar puncture and cisternal puncture methods. The most common imaging procedure that employs the intrathecal method is myelography.

TYPES OF CONTRAST MEDIA

IODINATED CONTRAST MEDIA

The iodine component of a modern contrast medium is able to absorb more radiation than the average tissues or organs of the body. When introduced into an organ or vessel, the iodine increases the opacity of the structure and can delineate the anatomical details of the organ or vessel on fluoroscopy or on a radiographic film and is therefore known as a positive or radiopaque contrast medium. Most types of iodinated contrast media used during radiological procedures today are water-based (water-soluble). A few radiological examinations use an oil-based (water-insoluble) iodinated contrast medium.

The oil-based iodinated contrast medium was developed for radiological examinations that require the contrast medium to persist during the procedure. For selected radiological examinations, rapid absorption of the contrast medium by the surrounding body tissues is undesirable. An oil-based contrast medium is not rapidly absorbed and does not easily mix with body fluids. Although oil-based contrast media are seldom used today, lymphangiography is an example of a radiological examination that still uses a water-insoluble contrast medium.

The various types of water-based iodinated contrast media are generally multipurpose agents that may be injected into organs or vessels. When injected into the patient's vessel, the contrast medium mixes with the blood and is eventually excreted by the kidneys. When an iodinated contrast medium is injected into an organ, the contrast medium is reabsorbed into the blood stream by the surrounding body tissues and is eventually excreted by the kidneys.

An important concept concerning radiographic contrast media is that in both cases, injecting the iodinated contrast medium directly into the blood stream or directly into an organ, the patient's urine will not be stained or discolored. A misconception that patients have about radiographic contrast media is that they are dyes. Most types of iodinated contrast media are colorless and are transparent to visible light. Their ability to enhance visualization of anatomical structures is due to the ability of contrast media to absorb radiation and not to its particular coloration.

Water-based radiographic contrast media may be supplied in ionic or non-ionic and monomer or dimer solutions. The specific characteristics of these solutions are determined by the number of particular molecules and the number and type of side chains attached to the basic iodine atoms. The use of a certain contrast medium is usually determined by the physician after careful consideration of the medical status of the patient. Table 6–1 is a summary of iodinated contrast media used in radiography.

GADOLINIUM-BASED CONTRAST MEDIUM

Iodine is used as the basis for injectable radiographic contrast media because of its ability to attenuate x-ray photons. Magnetic resonance imaging procedures do not use x-ray photons as a source of energy. A new class of contrast media for use during magnetic resonance imaging examinations has been developed. Gadolinium diethylenetriamine penta-acetic acid (Gd-DTPA) was developed as an injectable paramagnetic contrast medium for use during magnetic resonance imaging procedures. This contrast medium is capable of shortening the T1 and T2 relaxation times during a magnetic resonance scan, thus affecting the appearance of the image.

CHARACTERISTICS OF IODINATED CONTRAST MEDIA

The **chemical configuration** of injectable iodinated contrast media may be one of four types: ionic monomer, non-ionic monomer, ionic dimer, or non-ionic dimer. An ionic monomer iodinated contrast medium is configured by three iodine atoms (tri-iodinated) attached to a substituted benzoic acid ring derivative. Added to this ring structure is a cation such as sodium or meglumine; an anion radical such as diatrizoate, iothalamate, or metrizoate; and a carboxyl group (Fig. 6–1). When the iodinated contrast medium is placed in solution, such as blood, the carboxyl group causes a compound to be formed in which the anion and cation disassociate or dissolve. The ratio for the compound is the number of iodine atoms

TABLE 6–1

Summary of Iodinated Contrast Media Used in Radiography

Generic Name	Brand Name	Ionic Configuration	Relative Osmolality	Examples of Clinical Applications
Diatrizoate	Hypaque	Ionic monomer (3:2)	HOCM	Urography, vascular, multipurpose
Diatrizoate	Renografin	Ionic monomer (3:2)	HOCM	Multipurpose
Iodipamide	Cholografin	Ionic monomer (3:2)	HOCM	Intravenous cholangiography
Iophendylate	Pantopaque	Ionic monomer (3:2)	HOCM	Myelography
Iothalamate	Conray	Ionic monomer (3:2)	HOCM	Urography, vascular, multipurpose
Ethiodized oil	Ethiodol	Ionic monomer (3:2)	HOCM	Lymphography
Metrizamide	Amipaque	Non-ionic monomer (3:1)	HOCM	Myelography
Iohexol	Omnipaque	Non-ionic monomer (3:1)	HOCM	Myelography, vascular, multipurpose
Iopamidol	Isovue	Non-ionic monomer (3:1)	HOCM	Vascular
Ioversol	Optiray	Non-ionic monomer (3:1)	HOCM	Vascular
Iotrolan	Osmovist	Non-ionic dimer (6:1)	LOCM	
Ioxaglate	Hexabrix	Non-ionic dimer (6:1)	LOCM	Vascular, multipurpose

HOCM = high-osmolality contrast medium; LOCM = low-osmolality contrast medium.

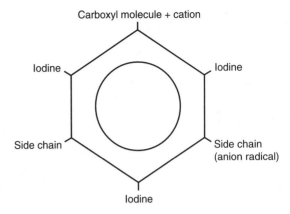

FIGURE 6-1
Chemical configuration of an ionic
monomer contrast medium.

to the number of particles (anion and cation) in solution. Ionic iodinated contrast
media are classified as $3:2$ compounds (numerical value of the ratio is 1.5, or
$3/2 = 1.5$) because they contain three atoms of iodine for each two particles (one
anion and one cation) in solution. In clinical practice, the meglumine-based agents
tend to be less toxic (see the following section on toxicity), but the sodium-based
agents tend to be less viscous (see the following section on viscosity). Hypaque
is an example of an ionic contrast medium.

An ionic dimer contrast medium molecule is based on the same benzoic acid
ring derivative. In this instance, two tri-iodinated benzoic acid rings are linked
together and share an ionizing radical (Fig. 6–2). Also, on one of the benzoic
acid rings, a non-ionizing amide is substituted for the carboxyl group, leaving only
one carboxyl group on the molecule. This type of contrast medium is classified
as a $6:2$ compound (numerical value of the ratio is 3) because it contains six
atoms of iodine to two particles in solution. The ionic dimer contrast media have
low osmolality (see the following section on osmolality) and tend to be less toxic

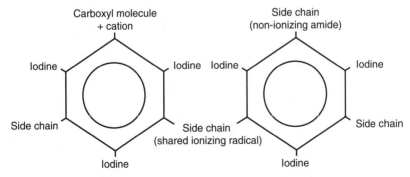

FIGURE 6-2
Chemical configuration of an ionic dimer contrast medium.

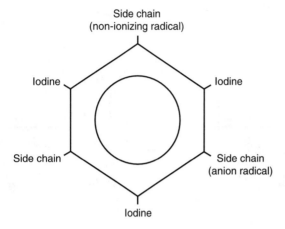

FIGURE 6–3
Chemical configuration of a non-ionic monomer contrast medium.

than the previously mentioned ionic agents, resulting in fewer side effects. Ioxaglate is an example of an ionic dimer contrast medium.

The recently developed non-ionic iodinated contrast media were also developed as a lower-osmolality alternative. The non-ionic monomer contrast medium has a basic structure consisting of a benzoic acid ring in which the carboxyl group is replaced with a non-ionizing side chain (Fig. 6–3). These non-ionic contrast media are classified as 3:1 compounds (numerical value of the ratio is 3) because they contain three iodine atoms to one particle of contrast medium in solution. Although these non-ionic contrast media tend to be expensive, their use in clinical practice has resulted in fewer adverse patient reactions. Iohexol, iopamidol, and ioversol are examples of non-ionic monomers.

The non-ionic dimer contrast medium consists of two non-ionic monomers attached to each other by an ionizing radical (Fig. 6–4). The result is six iodine atoms to one particle in solution. A 6:1 compound (numerical value of the ratio

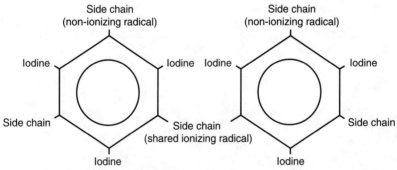

FIGURE 6–4
Chemical configuration of a non-ionic dimer contrast medium.

is 6) is obtained, which possesses lower osmolality than for a non-ionic monomer contrast medium. Iotrolan (Osmovist), iodecimol, and iodixanol are examples.

The **osmolality** of a contrast medium is determined by the number of particles in the solution. The osmolality of human blood is about 300 milliosmoles (mOsm) per kilogram (kg). Ionic contrast media have a minimum osmolality of 1000 mOsm/kg, and non-ionic contrast media have a minimum osmolality of 600 mOsm/kg. The osmolality for both types of contrast media is well above that for human blood. Thus, contrast media can penetrate blood cells. For example, an ionic contrast medium with a 3:2 chemical configuration has two osmolar particles, whereas a non-ionic contrast medium with a 3:1 chemical configuration has only one osmolar particle in solution. It is believed that a contrast medium with a lower osmolality (or higher numerical value of the ratio) is less toxic to the body tissues and thus produces fewer adverse patient reactions.

The **iodine concentration** of a contrast medium will determine its ability to absorb x-ray photons. For example, a contrast medium with a higher concentration of iodine will absorb more x-ray energy and is said to be more radiopaque. The amount of iodine and the concentration of iodine in the solution of a particular contrast medium can be determined from its label or from the product descriptive insert sheet. Iodine concentration is usually stated in units of milligrams per milliliter (mg/ml). Table 6–2 provides the approximate iodine content and osmolality of selected contrast media.

The **viscosity** of a solution such as a contrast medium is a measure of the resistance of the fluid to flow. Viscosity is determined by the number of particles in the solution and the attraction among these particles. A contrast medium with a high iodine concentration or with meglumine as its cation also tends to have a higher viscosity. A contrast medium with a high viscosity will require greater injection pressures for administration. Warming the contrast medium to body temperature (98.6° F) will reduce its viscosity and make it easier to inject.

The **toxicity** of a contrast medium on body tissues and organs is related to the contrast medium's chemical configuration, osmolality, iodine concentration, and rate of injection. Contrast media that are non-ionic, have a low osmolality

TABLE 6–2

Characteristics of Select Contrast Media

Name	Approximate Iodine Content (mg/ml)	Approximate Osmolality (mOsm/kg)
Diatrizoate	280	1500
Iothalamate	280	1500
Iohexol	300	700
Ioversol	320	700
Iopamidol	300	600
Ioxaglate	320	600

and low iodine concentration, and are injected slowly tend to be less toxic and produce fewer patient reactions or side effects.

When one is choosing an appropriate contrast medium, the final characteristic to consider is **cost**. The ionic contrast media, with their higher incidence of patient reactions, are less expensive. The newer non-ionic contrast media are much more expensive but tend to result in fewer patient reactions.

When a physician or institution is evaluating various injectable iodinated contrast media for use during radiological examinations, all of the previously mentioned characteristics must be considered in relation to the physical status of the patient.

PHARMACODYNAMICS AND PHARMACOKINETICS OF CONTRAST MEDIA

The pharmacodynamics and pharmacokinetics of contrast media are complex. This section presents a summary of pharmacodynamics and pharmacokinetics needed for the technologist to understand the effects contrast media have on the body, especially as they relate to adverse reactions (see Chapter 7, Preventive Care and Emergency Response to Contrast Media).

The primary factor in the production of adverse effects by contrast media is osmolality. Recall that the human body is composed mostly of water, and hemostasis is the body's ability to maintain proper balance of water. One method the body uses to maintain an appropriate water content is osmosis. In this method, water moves through a semipermeable membrane from an area of greater concentration to an area of lesser concentration. Because the osmolality of contrast media is greater than the body's osmolality, injection of contrast medium into the blood causes water to pass from the cells of the blood into the plasma and results in a shift of water from the extravascular area into the intravascular system. To maintain equilibrium, the contrast medium molecules diffuse from the plasma into the extracellular tissue. Contrast medium can enter all extracellular tissue through this process, except the vascular areas of the brain and testes, which limit the ability of fluids to move into tissues. As the contrast medium "washes out" of the blood, the new incoming blood results in a reversal of the osmotic pressure, and the movement of the water reverses. This movement of water and contrast medium results in adverse hemodynamic, erythrocyte, and capillary endothelium effects. This may manifest itself in the form of vasodilation, changes in blood volume (i.e., decrease in hematocrit), changes in pulmonary artery pressures, and alterations in cardiac output.

Another factor contributing to the toxicity of contrast media is the adverse effects of ionization. It is believed that the central nervous system is sensitive to ionic changes that interfere with the normal electrical activity of the body. When ionic contrast medium is introduced into the body, the medium dissociates and changes the ionic composition of the body. These ionic changes can result in seizures or cardiac dysfunction. Because non-ionic media do not produce adverse ionic changes, it is one reason to substitute ionic media with non-ionic agents.

The last factor that causes adverse response to contrast media is molecular toxicity. The molecular interaction of the contrast medium with the blood within the body has been recorded to result in histamine release, suppression of the activation of some enzymes, binding of the contrast agent to serum protein, increased thrombin time, increased coagulation time, and suppression of erythrocyte function. Non-ionic media have much less molecular toxicity than ionic media do.

CLINICAL APPLICATIONS

URINARY SYSTEM

Intravenous urography is a radiological examination of the urinary tract that includes the kidneys, ureters, and bladder. An intravenous injection of iodinated contrast medium is infused or given as a bolus. The contrast medium circulates throughout the blood stream and is eventually filtered out of the blood by the kidneys and is excreted. Contrast media tend to cause an initial vasodilation followed by vasoconstriction. The kidneys are responsible for eliminating the contrast medium from the body. In osmotic diuresis, the tubules fail to reabsorb the water and sodium. This results in dehydration of the patient. Contrast media with a numerical value of 3 (for the anion:cation ratio) decrease osmotic diuresis. Because of the adverse effects on the kidneys, it is important to check the function of the kidneys prior to contrast medium injection, e.g., by means of determination of the creatinine level. Diabetic and dehydrated patients are considered to be at high risk for harmful effects of contrast medium on the kidneys.

As the "iodine-loaded" urine flows from the kidneys to the bladder, the iodine can opacify the urinary structures. As the iodine absorbs radiation, it produces a white image of the anatomical details of the urinary system on the radiographic film. Some examples of contrast media used for urography include iothalamate (Conray), ioxaglate (Hexabrix), and diatrizoate (Hypaque or Renografin).

BILIARY SYSTEM

Cholangiography is a radiological examination of the biliary system following the intravenous injection of an iodinated contrast medium. An example of a contrast medium that has been used for intravenous cholangiography is iodipamide (Cholografin).

Today, fewer intravenous cholangiograms are performed. Endoscopic retrograde cholangiopancreatography (ERCP) is a more common imaging examination used to demonstrate the structures of the biliary tree. Endoscopic retrograde cholangiopancreatography uses a fiberoptic endoscope to demonstrate the anatomy of the common bile duct under fluoroscopic guidance. A contrast medium such as iohexol (Omnipaque) can be injected directly into the ductal system via the catheter in the endoscope.

SPINAL CORD

Myelography is a radiological examination of the spinal cord following the administration of a contrast medium into the subarachnoid space. The contrast medium is introduced into the subarachnoid space through a spinal needle via a lumbar or cisternal puncture. The oil-based iodinated contrast medium iophendylate (Pantopaque) was once used extensively for myelography. Metrizamide (Amipaque) was one of the first non-ionic, water-based contrast media developed and was used for myelography. Metrizamide is rarely used today for myelography because of reports of convulsions occurring when the contrast medium inadvertently reached the brain. Today, most physicians prefer to use one of the newer non-ionic, water-based iodinated contrast media such as iopamidol (Isovue) or iohexol (Omnipaque). These contrast media do not cross the blood-brain barrier, but they are able to mix with cerebrospinal fluid. Some adverse effects, such as seizures, mental changes, and aphasia, have been reported.

VASCULAR SYSTEM

Angiography, whether conventional or digital subtraction, is the radiological examination of a blood vessel following the administration of an iodinated contrast medium. Arteriography is the radiological examination of arterial structures, and venography is the radiological examination of venous structures. The blood vessel under investigation is usually approached through a catheter advanced from the femoral artery to the point of interest. The contrast medium is injected through the angiographic catheter. Ionic contrast media used for angiographic procedures include diatrizoate (Hypaque or Renografin) and iothalamate (Conray). Non-ionic contrast media used for angiographic procedures include iohexol (Omnipaque), iopamidol (Isovue), and ioversol (Optiray). These media have been known to cause vasodilation, increased blood flow, cardiac dysrhythmia, and blood pressure changes.

LYMPHATIC SYSTEM

Lymphography is the radiological examination of the lymphatic system following the administration of an oil-based contrast medium. The ethiodized oil Ethiodol is the oil-based contrast medium most commonly used for lymphographic examinations in the United States. This oil-based contrast medium is injected into a superficial lymphatic vessel on the top of the foot for demonstration of the lymphatic structures of the lower extremities and abdomen.

JOINTS

Arthrography is the radiological examination of the joint capsule and surrounding structures following the injection of an iodinated contrast medium. The articular surfaces of the joint along with the menisci are easily demonstrated on radiographic film following the injection of a contrast medium. The ionic diatrizoates (Hypaque and Renografin) can be used for arthrographic procedures. The newer non-ionic contrast media such as iopamidol (Isovue), iohexol (Omnipaque), and the low-osmolality agent ioxaglate (Hexabrix) are frequently used today for arthrography.

COMPUTED TOMOGRAPHY

Computed tomography examinations of the spinal cord may require the intrathecal administration of a non-ionic, water-based iodinated contrast medium. Many times a computed tomographic scan of the spinal cord is indicated following a myelogram. This postmyelogram computed tomographic study is usually scheduled 1–3 hours after the conventional myelogram, which allows for the contrast medium to be diluted by the patient's body so that it will not produce artifacts in the computed tomography images.

One can also perform a computed tomographic examination of the spinal cord structures without first performing a conventional myelogram. In this case, a low concentration of a non-ionic, iodinated contrast medium is introduced into the patient's subarachnoid space, and the scans are completed. Any of the non-ionic contrast media approved for intrathecal injections, such as iohexol or iopamidol, can be used for this procedure.

The use of an iodinated contrast medium during computed tomography studies of the rest of the body aids in detecting subtle lesions, demonstrating the blood supply to a mass, differentiating neoplastic processes from other abnormalities, and visualizing hepatic and biliary pathologies. Any of the contrast media approved for vascular or multipurpose uses can be injected intravenously for a computed tomographic study.

MAGNETIC RESONANCE IMAGING

In radiological procedures, iodine is administered as a contrast medium to enhance the visibility of anatomical details. In magnetic resonance imaging procedures, iodine is ineffective as a contrast medium. A paramagnetic contrast medium is used for magnetic resonance imaging procedures.

A paramagnetic contrast medium is a chemical that can alter the magnetic properties of body tissues. Because paramagnetic substances have an abundance of unpaired electrons in their atoms, they are able to generate a strong magnetic field that results in shortening of the T1 and T2 relaxation times. Gadolinium is an element with unpaired electrons and is an effective contrast enhancer for magnetic resonance imaging.

Gadolinium, however, is highly toxic to humans. To modify its toxicity, a chelated metal complex is combined with the gadolinium. The most common chelate used is diethylenetriamine penta-acetic acid (DTPA).

Gadolinium–diethylenetriamine penta-acetic acid (Gd-DTPA) may be injected via the intravenous, intra-arterial, or intrathecal route. It is effective in diagnosing disk disease and scar tissue in the vertebral column. It is also effective for the diagnosis of infarction, tumors, vascular lesions, and demyelinating diseases.

PRECAUTIONS

ADVERSE EFFECTS ASSOCIATED WITH IONIC CONTRAST MEDIA

The injection of an ionic iodinated contrast medium may lead to adverse effects. It is thought that these adverse reactions are related to the osmolality of the contrast medium. The use of the new low-osmolality contrast media tends to result in fewer and less severe adverse effects. The expense, however, of these low-osmolality contrast media has resulted in many institutions' still stocking and using the older ionic media.

During injection of an ionic contrast medium, the patient may experience a warm feeling throughout his or her body. Pain at the injection site may indicate extravasation of the contrast medium into surrounding tissues.

Some patients may experience light-headedness, nausea, vomiting, or urticarial patches. These effects usually are short-lived.

More serious complications of hypotension, bronchospasm, dysrhythmia, and laryngeal edema may occur. These complications require immediate medical intervention. Common anaphylactoid reactions to radiographic contrast media are described in detail in Chapter 7.

PEDIATRIC IMAGING

According to the contrast medium product descriptive insert sheet, the dosage of an iodinated contrast medium administered to pediatric patients for radiological imaging procedures is usually based on patient weight. The usual dosage rate is calculated at 1 ml/kg of the patient's body weight for pelvic computed tomography; 2 ml/kg for intravenous pyelography and computed tomography of the chest and abdomen; and up to 6 ml/kg for angiography. Digital subtraction angiography, however, utilizes a half-strength dilution of the contrast medium.

Because of their increased safety, the new non-ionic or low-osmolality iodinated contrast media are preferred for intravenous, intra-arterial, or intrathecal injections during pediatric radiological procedures. Although the use of the new non-ionic and low-osmolality contrast media tends to result in fewer adverse reactions, their injection for pediatric imaging is not without risk. A physician, therefore, should be immediately available throughout the radiological procedure when a parenteral injection of an iodinated contrast medium is indicated.

PATIENT HISTORY

A thorough patient history taken prior to the injection of an iodinated contrast medium may indicate conditions that would place the patient at a higher risk for adverse reactions. Many physicians and institutions will administer a low-osmolality contrast medium to these patients in order to reduce the incidence and severity of complications.

Patients who have experienced a previous adverse reaction to an iodinated contrast medium injection or who have experienced previous general allergic episodes are more likely to have an adverse side effect from the contrast medium injection. Patients with a history of asthma are particularly at risk.

Other patient characteristics that may indicate the need for a low-osmolality contrast medium include age (infants and the aged), heart disease, severe diabetes, multiple myeloma, and renal insufficiency.

BIBLIOGRAPHY

Abrams HT (ed): Abrams angiography: vascular and interventional radiology, 3rd edition. Little, Brown, Boston, 1983.

Amiel M (ed): Contrast media in radiology. Springer-Verlag, Berlin, 1982.

Ballinger PW: Merrill's atlas of radiographic positions and radiological procedures, 7th edition. Mosby-Year Book, St. Louis, 1991.

Grossman W, Baim DS: Cardiac catheterization, angiography, and intervention, 4th edition. Lea & Febiger, Philadelphia, 1991.

Ehrlich RA, McCloskey ED: Patient care in radiography. Mosby-Year Book, St. Louis, 1993.

Katzberg, RW (ed): The contrast media manual. Williams & Wilkins, Baltimore, 1992.

Kruger RA, Riederer SJ: Basic concepts of digital subtraction angiography. GK Hall Medical Publishers, Boston, 1984.

Parvez Z, Moncada R, Sovak M: Contrast media: biological effects and clinical application. CRC Press, Boca Raton, FL, 1987.

Skucas, J: Radiographic contrast agents, 2nd edition. Aspen Publishers, Rockville, MD, 1989.

Snopek AM: Fundamentals of special radiographic procedures, 3rd edition. WB Saunders, Philadelphia, 1992.

Tortorici MR: Fundamentals of angiography. CV Mosby, St. Louis, 1982.

Preventive Care and Emergency Response to Contrast Medium Reactions

JOSEPH R. BITTENGLE, M.Ed., ARRT(R)
DONNA C. DAVIS, M.Ed., ARRT(R)(CV)

7

INTRODUCTION

The administration of radiological contrast medium to patients is almost as old as the discovery of x-rays. Over the years, many cases of adverse reactions to contrast media have been documented. Numerous studies have been performed to determine the cause of the reactions in hopes of finding drugs to reverse the reaction. Although major advancements have been made in the production of contrast media, the perfect medium has yet to be discovered. However, some success has been attained in reducing the number and intensity of reactions.

This chapter discusses common preprocedural care protocols used to decrease the number and intensity of reactions. It also identifies the various types of reactions that tend to occur in patients. It further discusses common treatment for the various reactions as well as recommended postprocedural care.

PATIENT EDUCATION AND ASSESSMENT

The ability of the imaging technologist to communicate effectively with a patient is paramount in properly preparing the patient for an imaging procedure that requires the injection of a radiopaque contrast medium. The primary goals of this one-on-one communication include gaining the cooperation of the patient during the procedure, informing the patient about the impending procedure, answering any questions the patient may have, allaying any anxiety the patient may be experiencing, and assisting in obtaining an informed consent for the imaging procedure.

PROVIDING PROCEDURAL INFORMATION

Effective interpersonal communication skills on the part of the imaging technologist are an important aspect of gaining the cooperation of the patient. A thorough explanation of the procedure and the patient's role during the procedure usually alleviates apprehension and anxiety. A well-informed and relaxed patient tends to enhance the performance of the imaging procedure.

While informing the patient about the imaging procedure, the technologist should include the following: the purpose of the procedure, how the procedure will be carried out, the expected duration of the procedure, and any limitations or restrictions associated with the procedure. The reasons for ordering the procedure should be fully explained to the patient. A thorough description of the procedural methods should also be provided. It is important to avoid using technical terms when explaining the procedure. To help ensure that the patient understands what is being said, the technologist should use "lay" terms. Also, an opportunity for the patient to ask questions should be encouraged. The anticipated duration of the procedure should be provided, especially for geriatric patients, whose sense of security, control, and orientation may be enhanced by this information. It is also appropriate to "remind" the patient of procedural methods, time duration, etc., during the procedure. Finally, any limitations in the efficacy of the procedure or any restrictions placed on the patient following the procedure should be fully explained. If the procedure requires restrictions, it is advisable to submit them in writing to the patient in addition to verbally explaining them. If the patient is medicated, this process should be repeated for a relative or other responsible person who can care for the patient.

ANXIETY FACTORS

The imaging technologist must be aware of several possible preconceived notions the patient may have that may produce anxiety and hinder the imaging technologist's ability to effectively communicate with the patient. For example, some patients assume that the imaging procedure is performed only in seriously or critically ill patients. This belief can hinder all attempts to provide rational explanations about the procedure and obstruct cooperation on the part of the patient. Other patients may exhibit a fear of the unknown. Still others may have received false information about the procedure from friends or family members. For example, a patient may believe that the x-ray "dye" will stain the urine. The imaging technologist must assess the knowledge and beliefs of the patient to gain a better understanding of the patient's feelings. This information may be obtained by asking open-ended questions, such as "What do you know about this procedure?" Through a gentle, personable approach and by providing accurate information, answering patient questions, and projecting the image of a competent, compassionate care giver, the technologist should be able to allay any anxieties of the patient.

COMMUNICATION

Communication with the patient must be at a level that is understandable to the patient. The imaging technologist's selection of terminology and explanations must be tempered by the perceived intelligence level of the patient, the patient's own communication and language skills, and the patient's level of consciousness. Communication with the patient is the opportunity to create a favorable "first impression." The goal is to provide an image of a caring and competent technologist.

INFORMED CONSENT

The imaging technologist is responsible for ensuring that the patient has signed an informed consent form. This form should be designed to advise the patient of what procedure has been ordered, the methods or techniques that will be used to complete the procedure, the benefits and risks of the procedure, and any alternative procedures that may be available.

Informed consent forms prepared by medical facilities may appear different. Most radiological informed consent forms generally address several topics, however. These include an authorization paragraph, a disclosure paragraph, a nonguarantee paragraph, a patient understanding paragraph, and a place for signatures. The authorization clause identifies the facility and people who will be performing the procedure. Explanation of the procedure and descriptions of benefits and risks and of alternative examinations are in the disclosure statement. The nonguarantee statement is a simple sentence indicating that there is no guarantee of results associated with the procedure. The patient understanding statement indicates that the content of the form was discussed with the patient and that the patient agrees to undergo the procedure. The discussion of the contents of the form is the responsibility of the physician, *not* the technologist. Also, time for patient questions should be provided and encouraged. Table 7–1 is a representative consent form for radiological contrast medium procedures.

PATIENT PREPARATION

In assessing a patient's physical and emotional preparation for an imaging procedure, several steps should be followed prior to the procedure. In preparation for the procedure, the imaging technologist should verify the patient's identity, greet the patient respectfully, and introduce himself or herself. The imaging technologist should verify the written order for the procedure and that all preprocedural orders have been carried out. This information is located in the patient's chart. Example preprocedural orders include fasting for 6–8 hours before the procedure or a restriction to clear fluids, establishing access and hydration, and documenting baseline vital signs prior to administration of any premedication. It is the responsibility of the physician to determine which current routine medications should be given on the day of the procedure and which medications should be withheld. For example, with a patient scheduled for a coronary arteriogram, anticoagulation therapy may have to be discontinued prior to the procedure. Besides verifying the written orders, the technologist should review the patient's chart to determine the patient's medical history. The status of the patient's renal function, bleeding tendencies (e.g., sickle cell anemia), current medications, and previous contrast medium reactions influence how, or if, the procedure should be performed.

Other items of the patient's medical history that should be documented include any cardiac arrhythmias or blood pressure instability and the patient's allergy history. The imaging technologist should also review laboratory values for prothrombin time (PT), partial thromboplastin time (PTT and APTT), hematocrit, blood urea nitrogen (BUN), and creatinine (Table 7–2). These tests assess the clotting ability of blood, the function of the kidneys, and liver performance.

Prior to any contrast medium injection, the vital signs of the patient should be measured and documented. These vital signs should include heart rate, blood pressure, respiration rate, and blood oxygen saturation. In the case of angiography,

TABLE 7–1

Informed Consent for Radiological Contrast Medium Procedures

Name_____ Date_____ Time_____ a.m./p.m.
Referring Physician_____ Radiologist_____
Procedure_____
  I have been informed that this radiological contrast medium procedure listed above may require the use of needles, catheters, local anesthesia, radiological contrast media (x-ray dye), or various medications and solutions. Possible alternative methods to this procedure have been explained to me.
  I have been informed that this radiological contrast medium procedure listed above will provide valuable diagnostic information. I have also been informed that this radiological contrast medium procedure listed above also carries some risk. I understand that these risks may include: bleeding; infection; damage to adjacent tissues; swelling; allergic reaction; renal, pulmonary, or cardiac failure; or cerebral complications. I have also been informed that surgery may be necessary to correct these complications.
  I recognize that the results of this radiological contrast medium procedure cannot be guaranteed.
  I have read (or have had it read to me in a language understandable to me) this consent form, understand its contents, have had an opportunity to ask questions, and have had all my questions answered. I hereby give my consent for the performance of this radiological contrast medium procedure on me. I also consent to the administration of premedications and/or local anesthetics as may be necessary in the performance of this radiological contrast medium procedure. I also consent to the performance of any emergency procedures deemed appropriate by the radiologist to correct any complications that may arise. I assume all risks and complications associated with this radiological contrast medium procedure listed above.
Signature_____ (Patient/authorized legal guardian)
Relationship of guardian to patient _____
Witness Signature_____ Date_____
  I have explained this radiological contrast medium procedure to the patient and any risks or complications associated with this procedure. The patient has indicated his/her understanding of this radiological contrast medium procedure and has given consent for the performance of this procedure.
Radiologist's Signature_____ Date_____

depending on the nature of the procedure, pulses should be recorded for the right and left radial arteries, right and left femoral arteries, and the right and left dorsalis pedis arteries. The patient should also be assessed for any risk factors for adverse reactions to the contrast medium injection (Table 7–3). The availability of a well-stocked, up-to-date crash cart must be assured. Table 7–4 is a summary of the preprocedural patient preparation protocol.

PREMEDICATION

Premedication protocols vary among physicians, medical facilities, and imaging procedures. Protocols also vary with patient age, patient weight, current medica-

TABLE 7-2

Summary of Laboratory Values

Test Name	Purpose	Normal Values	Critical Values	Possible Indications of Abnormal Value
Activated partial thromboplastin time (APTT or PTT)	Assess intrinsic blood coagulation system	27–38 sec	>100 sec or <25 sec	Clotting factor deficiencies, cirrhosis, leukemia, hemophilia, disseminated intravascular coagulation
Prothrombin time (PT)	Assess extrinsic blood clotting mechanism	9–13 sec	>19 sec or <8 sec	Cirrhosis, hepatitis, disseminated intravascular coagulation
Blood urea nitrogen (BUN)	Assess metabolic function of the liver and excretory function of the kidneys	6–20 mg/dl	—	Renal disease, renal failure, hypovolemia, congestive heart failure, myocardial infarction, dehydration
Serum creatnine	Assess renal excretory function	0.5–1.1 mg/dl	—	Renal disease, diabetes mellitus
Hematocrit (Hct)	Assess percentage of red blood cells in total blood volume	34–50%	>55% or <21%	Anemia, cirrhosis, hemolytic reaction, hemorrhage, bone marrow failure, multiple myeloma, leukemia

TABLE 7–3

Risk Factors for Reactions to Contrast Medium Injection

Asthma and allergies
Cardiovascular disease (coronary artery disease)
Cirrhosis
Dehydration
Diabetes mellitus
Elderly
Hepatic disease
Hypertension
Increased intracranial pressure
Metastatic cancer
Multiple chronic illnesses
Pediatric patients
Peripheral vascular disease
Previous contrast medium injection
Previous contrast medium reaction
Primary cancer
Renal disease
Respiratory disease (chronic obstructive pulmonary disease)
Sickle cell anemia

tions, overall health, and whether the patient is known to be at risk for an allergic reaction.

A typical premedication protocol for a nonallergic patient may include the administration of a mild sedative such as diazepam (Valium), lorazepam (Ativan), hydroxyzine HCl (Vistaril), or alprazolam (Xanax). The purpose of a mild sedative is to help reduce the patient's anxiety level. One of these sedatives is usually administered to the patient undergoing more complex, invasive angiographic procedures and is probably not normally indicated for a patient undergoing intravenous urography.

A typical protocol for patients with a known allergic history may include the administration of diphenhydramine HCl (Benadryl). Diphenhydramine is an antihistamine and reduces the possible incidence of contrast medium reactions. Additionally, corticosteroid preparations, such as methylprednisolone (Solu-Medrol), dexamethasone (Decadron), or prednisone (Deltasone), may be given. Corticosteroids are indicated in the treatment of chronic or acute inflammatory disorders. Cimetidine (Tagamet) may also be administered to reduce the secretion of gastric juices. Table 7–5 is a summary of common premedication protocols.

All premedication protocols must be adjusted according to the patient's age, weight, physical condition, medical and allergic histories, and drug or alcohol abuse history. Table 7–3 lists several risk factors that must be considered prior to the administration of any premedication.

TABLE 7–4

Summary of Preprocedural Patient Preparation Protocol

1. Check patient identification, greet patient, identify self
2. Verify preprocedural orders
3. Explain procedure
4. Answer patient's questions
5. Review patient's medical history
6. Review patient's allergy history
7. Obtain baseline vital signs
8. Assess patient's risk factors
9. Verify availability of crash cart

Following the administration of any premedication, the patient's heart rate, blood pressure, respiration rate, blood oxygen saturation, and changes in the level of consciousness should be monitored. When a significant deviation of these values from the patient's baseline values occurs, the physician should be summoned immediately. All incidents of a patient's adverse reaction to premedication should be accurately and promptly documented (see Chapter 10, Documentation).

TABLE 7–5

Common Premedication Protocols

Drug	Classification	Dose	Action
diazepam (Valium)	Antianxiety	10 mg oral	Reduces anxiety
lorazepam (Ativan)	Antianxiety	1 mg intravenous	Reduces anxiety
hydroxyzine HCl (Vistaril)	Antianxiety	50–100 mg oral	Reduces anxiety
alprazolam (Xanax)	Antianxiety	0.25–0.5 mg oral	Reduces anxiety
diphenhydramine HCl (Benadryl)	Antihistamine	50 mg oral, intravenous, or intramuscular	Reduces release of histamine
methylprednisolone (Solu-Medrol)	Corticosteroid	30 mg intravenous	Reduces inflammatory responses
dexamethasone (Decadron)	Corticosteroid	6–10 mg intravenous	Reduces inflammatory responses
prednisone (Deltasone)	Corticosteroid	50 mg oral (3 times)	Reduces inflammatory responses
cimetidine (Tagamet)	Antiulcer	300 mg intravenous (with normal saline)	Reduces gastric secretion

TYPES OF CONTRAST MEDIUM REACTIONS

Anaphylactoid or idiosyncratic reactions to an iodinated contrast medium range in severity from minor to intermediate to major. Minor adverse contrast medium reactions may progress to an intermediate or major response and tend to be unpredictable.

Reactions to an iodinated contrast medium cannot be reliably predicted by utilizing a skin test dose. A person who received an injection of an iodinated contrast medium and who experienced no adverse reaction may still experience adverse side effects on a subsequent contrast medium administration. Conversely, a patient who received an iodinated contrast medium injection and who did experience an adverse side effect may experience no reaction after receiving a second injection. However, previous adverse reactions associated with the administration of an iodinated contrast medium are still considered a risk factor that most physicians will recognize as requiring caution and a preventive premedication protocol.

Most reactions occur following an intravascular injection of relatively large doses of an iodinated contrast medium during such radiological procedures as intravenous urography and angiography. Higher rates of reaction seem to follow intravenous injections as opposed to intra-arterial injections. Patients with prior allergies to certain foods or pollens are approximately twice as likely to experience a contrast medium reaction. Asthmatic patients are approximately three times more likely to experience adverse side effects than nonasthmatic patients. Likewise, those who have had a previous reaction to contrast medium are approximately three times more likely to experience another adverse response. Severe contrast medium reactions occur in approximately 1 of every 14,000 cases. Fatal contrast medium reactions occur in 1 of every 40,000 cases. Patient characteristics that tend to increase the mortality rate include age greater than 50 years, pre-existing cardiopulmonary disease, existing hypotension, and alcoholism.

Although the cause of adverse reactions to an iodinated contrast medium is unknown, some theories have been postulated. These theories tend to center on the liberation of histamine and complement (a serum enzyme protein). In the proximity of a foreign molecule approximately the size of six amino acids or larger, mast cells (connective tissue cells whose specific physiological function is unknown) in the body release histamine. This histamine release can cause an increase in vascular permeability and smooth muscle contraction. The various types of contrast media are also known to directly induce mast cell degranulation. Ionic contrast media tend to cause a release of more histamines and result in greater complement activation than non-ionic contrast media.

Complement is capable of producing lytic changes in the blood in response to an antigen-antibody reaction. These lytic changes result in red blood cell hemolysis, crenation (formation of abnormal notching), and sickling. Anaphylatoxin, a complement substance, promotes vessel permeability and the resultant increase in edema formation.

GENERALIZED EFFECTS

As a foreign substance, radiological contrast medium may cause recognizable effects when it is injected into the human body. These effects include toxic effects, osmolar effects, and allergic effects.

The chemotoxicity of the iodine atom is related to its ability to bind to protein molecules, resulting in an altered metabolism of the endothelium. Clinical manifestations of this toxic effect are nausea, vomiting, gastrointestinal edema, and seizures.

The osmolar effect of the iodinated contrast medium results in a shift in intracellular water and a disruption of vessel transport hemostasis. Water is transferred through the cellular membrane in the presence of high-osmolality solutions. Clinical symptoms of pain, heat (warmth), hypotension, and ventricular tachycardia are associated with this hyperosmolality characteristic of a radiological contrast medium.

The allergic effect represents an individual's unique physiological response to the contrast medium. Whereas the majority of patients generally experience no allergic response to an iodinated contrast medium injection, an idiosyncratic response in some individuals is unpredictable.

Common transient sensations associated with the intravascular administration of an iodinated contrast medium include warmth, flushing, and metallic taste. Although these sensations are typically not classified as adverse reactions, it is important to inform the patient of their possible occurrence and to reassure the patient that these are common and transient. In most cases, no medical intervention is indicated.

VASOVAGAL REACTIONS

Vasovagal reactions are associated with cardiovascular changes manifested in response to a contrast medium injection. Vasovagal reactions may be triggered by emotional and/or psychological stimuli. Cardiac electrical conduction alterations, namely, changes in both the sinoatrial and the atrioventricular nodal activity, have been documented. The resultant increase in peripheral vasodilation of arterioles, thought to be a result of the contrast medium osmolality, can lead to symptoms such as lightheadedness, anxiety, diaphoresis, systemic hypotension, and sinus bradycardia. The imaging technologist is advised that a progressive drop in systemic blood pressure can result in a loss of consciousness and a life-threatening situation. Vasovagal reactions are generally treated by placing the patient in the Trendelenburg position, initiating fluid replacement, and administering atropine in cases of sinus bradycardia.

ANAPHYLACTOID AND IDIOSYNCRATIC REACTIONS

There are several types of anaphylactoid reactions. These include cutaneous, gastrointestinal, central nervous system, respiratory, and cardiovascular responses.

The types of reactions in each of these areas are summarized below. Table 7–6 is a summary of the minor, intermediate, and major reactions associated with these areas. Table 7–7 summarizes common drug therapies for contrast media reactions.

Cutaneous Responses

Cutaneous responses to intravascular injections of an iodinated contrast medium are generally minor. Minor cutaneous responses may include mild urticaria, itching, pallor, and mild angioedema. It is important to note that urticarial reactions may occur within minutes to hours after an injection of a contrast medium. These mild responses are generally self-limiting and require no medical intervention. Moderate, nonresponsive urticaria and advancing angioedema are generally classified as intermediate cutaneous responses. The medications of choice for treatment of these intermediate cutaneous responses include diphenhydramine HCl (Benadryl) and epinephrine (Adrenalin).

TABLE 7–6

Minor, Intermediate, and Major Anaphylactoid Reactions of Systems

System	Minor Reactions	Intermediate Reactions	Major Reactions
Cutaneous	Mild urticaria Itching Pallor Mild angioedema	Moderate nonresponsive urticaria Moderate angioedema	None
Gastrointestinal	Nausea Vomiting	Severe vomiting Diarrhea Abdominal cramping	None
Central nervous	Headache Dizziness	Aphasia Amblyopia	Seizure Paresis Unconsciousness Coma
Respiratory	Sneezing Wheezing Coughing Rhinorrhea	Mild dyspnea Mild pulmonary edema Mild bronchospasm	Severe dyspnea Cyanosis Severe pulmonary edema Severe bronchospasm Laryngospasm Epiglottitis Respiratory arrest
Cardiovascular	Tachycardia	Mild hypotension Thready pulse Bradycardia	Acute severe hypotension Cardiac dysrhythmias Loss of consciousness Cardiac arrest

TABLE 7-7

Common Drug Therapies for Treatment of Contrast Medium Reactions

Drug	Classification	Dose	Route of Administration	Action
atropine sulfate	Anticholinergic	0.6–1.0 mg	Slow intravenous	Increases heart rate
diphenhydramine HCl (Benadryl)	Antihistamine	25–50 mg	Oral, intravenous, or intramuscular	Relieves allergic responses
epinephrine (Adrenalin)	Bronchodilator	0.1–0.3 ml (1:1000) 1.0–3.0 ml (1:10,000)	Subcutaneous or Intravenous	Increases blood pressure, relaxes bronchioles, increases heart rate, vasoconstrictor
promethazine HCl (Phenergan)	Antihistamine	12.5–25 mg	Oral or intravenous	Relieves nausea, relieves vomiting
furosemide (Lasix)	Diuretic	40 mg	Slow intravenous	Increases urine output
metaproterenol sulfate (Alupent)	Bronchodilator	2–3	Inhalation	Relaxes bronchioles
theophylline ethylenediamine (Aminophylline)	Bronchodilator	6.0 mg/kg	Intravenous with D5W over 20 minutes, then 0.4–1.0 mg/kg/hr as required	Relaxes bronchioles
diazepam (Valium)	Antianxiety	5–10 mg	Intravenous	Mild sedative

Gastrointestinal Responses

Mild nausea and vomiting are generally classified as minor gastrointestinal responses. These are common occurrences in patients who did not follow the customary preprocedural fasting orders or in patients who are in need of an emergency radiological examination requiring a contrast medium injection. These responses tend to be self-limiting and generally require no medical intervention, although an emesis basin should be provided for the patient. Additionally, to avoid aspiration, the patient should be adjusted into the right lateral position. Severe vomiting, diarrhea, intestinal edema, and abdominal cramping are additional adverse gastrointestinal responses. The administration of oxygen via a nasal cannula or of promethazine HCl (Phenergan), or both, tends to relieve mild cases of nausea and vomiting.

Central Nervous System Responses

Minor central nervous system responses may include headache and dizziness. Intermediate responses include aphasia and amblyopia. These minor and intermediate responses tend to be self-limiting, though at times they can be distressful to the patient. Major central nervous system responses may include seizures, paresis, unconsciousness, and coma. Seizures are thought to be associated with the iodinated contrast medium's ability to disrupt the blood-brain barrier. Seizures have also been associated in patients with primary or secondary metastatic cerebral lesions who have undergone contrast medium–enhanced radiological procedures. Generally, the treatment indicated for seizures includes no intervention except ensuring patient safety, unless the seizures are recurrent. Typical treatment protocols for seizures or convulsions may include oxygen administration, diazepam (Valium) administration, and monitoring vital signs as required.

Respiratory Responses

Minor respiratory responses may include sneezing, wheezing, coughing, and rhinorrhea. Like all minor reactions, any of these respiratory responses can progress to an intermediate or major response, though they tend to be self-limiting and generally require no treatment. Intermediate respiratory effects may include mild dyspnea, mild pulmonary edema, and mild bronchospasm. The administration of nasal oxygen, epinephrine (Adrenalin), and a diuretic such as furosemide (Lasix) and the placement of the patient in the Fowler position may be indicated. Major respiratory manifestations that may lead to a life-threatening situation include severe dyspnea, cyanosis, severe pulmonary edema, severe bronchospasm, laryngospasm, epiglottitis, and respiratory arrest. Additional drugs that may be indicated include metaproterenol sulfate (Alupent) and theophylline ethylenediamine (Aminophylline). If the patient's oxygen saturation falls below 89%, the emergency response team (code team) should be summoned.

Cardiovascular Responses

Tachycardia, a common anxiety-related response seen in patients undergoing a contrast medium injection, is generally classified as a minor cardiovascular reaction. This response is generally alleviated by a calm reassuring demeanor on the part of the imaging technologist. Intermediate cardiovascular responses include mild hypotension, thready pulse, and bradycardia. Treatment measures may include placing the patient in the Trendelenburg position, administration of nasal oxygen, intravenous fluid replacement, and the administration of atropine sulfate (Atropine). Major, life-threatening cardiovascular responses include acute severe hypotension, cardiac dysrhythmias, loss of consciousness, and cardiac arrest. The astute imaging technologist must be able to differentiate between hypotension with tachycardia and hypotension with bradycardia, because treatment protocols are different for each response. The treatment for hypotension with tachycardia usually includes the administration of epinephrine (Adrenalin) and fluid replacement, whereas the treatment of hypotension with bradycardia usually includes the administration of atropine sulfate (Atropine) and fluid replacement. In instances of full cardiac arrest, the imaging technologist must be prepared to initiate life-saving procedures such as CPR and to summon the code team.

RENAL EFFECTS

Intravascular injections of an iodinated contrast medium can produce physiological effects in the kidneys. Alterations in blood flow and glomerular activity may occur, resulting in diuresis.

Renal toxicity is a direct result of damage to the renal parenchyma. Of particular importance is the assessment of the patient's serum creatinine laboratory values. With creatinine values exceeding 2 mg/dl, the majority of renal complications can be reversed with adequate hydration. A creatinine level of 5 mg/dl may result in irreversible renal damage in the majority of patients who receive a contrast medium injection. Acute renal failure, whether oliguric (less fluid output than input) or non-oliguric, is a possible complication.

Patients with a heightened risk of renal-associated responses include those with prior renal disease, the elderly, those with diabetes, and those experiencing dehydration. Other risk factors include multiple myeloma, plasmacytoma, and increased uric acid concentrations. Patients with known pheochromocytoma, an adrenal gland tumor, may experience additional hypertensive episodes following administration of an iodinated contrast medium. In these hypertensive crises, it is the imaging technologist's responsibility to relate to the physician an accurate assessment of the patient's baseline status versus the patient's current post-injection status.

POSTPROCEDURAL CARE

Several factors influence the type of follow-up care provided after an injection of iodinated contrast medium. It is important to note that regardless of the situation, commonalities among postprocedural care protocols should include monitoring the vital signs of the patient, encouraging increased fluid intake, and orders to contact the physician if the patient's status changes. Postprocedural orders relative to an outpatient intravenous urogram may include the following: encouraging fluid intake, observing the patient, and orders to call the physician if the patient's status changes. An example of postprocedural orders for an inpatient angiogram via the femoral artery might include compression of the injection site for 10 minutes (15–20 minutes in hypertensive patients); immobilization of the extremity for 6–8 hours; checking the puncture site for internal and external bleeding; checking distal pulses and vital signs four times an hour for the first 4 hours, then two times an hour for the next 4 hours, and then every hour for the next 4 hours; assessing the entry extremity for temperature, color, and sensory responses; administering approximately 200 ml of intravenous fluid; encouraging oral fluid intake; reinstituting regular diet; and contacting the physician if complications arise.

The imaging technologist must document patient characteristics, changes in patient status, and any reaction before, during, and after the procedure (see Chapter 10, Documentation). Specifically, the following information should be charted by either the imaging technologist or the physician: the time the procedure began and ended, the contrast medium type, the route of administration, the amount used, the time the injection was made and the type of needle used, the patient's tolerance of the procedure, any adverse reaction, any medical intervention, patient instructions, and postprocedural orders.

BIBLIOGRAPHY

Adler, AM, and Carlton, M: Introduction to radiography and patient care. WB Saunders, Philadelphia, 1994.

Bush, WH, and Swanson, DP: Acute reactions to intravascular contrast media: types, risk factors, recognition and specific treatment. Am J Roentgenol 157:1153, 1991.

Campese, VM, et al: Contrast induced acute renal failure. Adv Exp Med Biol 212:135, 1987.

Greenberger, PA, and Patterson, R: The prevention of immediate generalized reactions to radiocontrast media in high-risk patients. J Allergy Clin Immunol 87:867, 1991.

Katayama, H, Yamaguchi, K, and Kozuka, T, et al: Adverse reactions to ionic and nonionic contrast media. Radiology 175:621, 1990.

Laudicina, P, and Wean, D: Applied angiography for radiographers. WB Saunders, Philadelphia, 1994.

Pagana, KD, and Pagana, TJ: Mosby's diagnostic and laboratory test reference. Mosby-Year Book, St. Louis, 1992.

Physicians Desk Reference, 49th edition. Medical Economics Data Production Company, Montvale, NJ, 1995.

Snopek, AM: Fundamentals of special radiographic procedures. WB Saunders, Philadelphia, 1992.

Imaging Pharmaceutical Compatibility

8

Introduction
Research Studies Regarding Contrast
   Media
Factors That May Influence
   Radiopharmaceutical Localization

INTRODUCTION

The most common type of pharmaceuticals that technologists are most apt to use are contrast media and radiopharmaceuticals. However, the technologist can expect to come in contact with other drugs. These can be divided in three categories: drugs used for emergencies, e.g., cardiac arrest, contrast medium reaction; preprocedural pharmaceuticals; and medications used to improve the diagnostic or therapeutic procedure results. In many instances, the technologist's job is to assist with administration of the drug, rather than administer the medication. Some of the drugs are administered within the imaging department, whereas others may be administered outside the department. Drugs administered within the department are of most concern because they would be most apt to be mixed with contrast media and cause an adverse reaction. Pharmaceuticals commonly employed in imaging or therapy include antihistamines, antibiotics, anticoagulants, sedatives, vasoconstrictors, and vasodilators.

This chapter contains information regarding the incompatibility of drugs with contrast media and the effect of mixing radiopharmaceuticals with medications. It should be noted that because new medications are constantly evolving, some of the drugs mentioned in this chapter may already have been replaced with newer, more modern medications.

RESEARCH STUDIES REGARDING CONTRAST MEDIA

Inpatients entering the imaging department commonly have an intravenous infusion access device in place. It is common practice for these access devices to be used to inject a contrast medium and other medications. Sometimes the contrast medium may precipitate if it comes in contact with any residual from another medication. A precipitate can cause a thrombus or embolus. Thus, it is important to know what medications are compatible or incompatible with various contrast media. One method to avoid an adverse reaction from incompatible medications is to flush the venous or arterial access device before and after the administration of contrast medium. The ability to inject a contrast medium depends on the type of medication in the access device, because the contrast medium may chemically react with the drug. Because of the thousands of drugs available in the United States, it is impossible to assess all of them for their compatibility with the numerous contrast media available. However, several studies have tested the compatibility of contrast media with other medications. The following is a summary of some of these investigations.

One study performed by Pilla and coworkers mixed 1 ml of undiluted papaverine hydrochloride (HCl) with 3 ml each of Renografin 76 (diatrizoate meglumine), Amipaque (metrizamide), and Conray 60 (iothalamate meglumine). Other tests included diluting papaverine HCl to various degrees and mixing each dilution with 5 ml Hexabrix (ioxaglate meglumine). Additionally, a 10 : 1 dilution of papaverine HCl was mixed with 15 and 30 ml of Hexabrix. Also, a 20 : 1 dilution was mixed with 5 ml of Hexabrix. Pilla and associates demonstrated that Renografin 76 developed a white suspension that disappeared. Conray 60 and Amipaque were able to mix with papaverine HCl with no response. Hexabrix precipitated immediately except when the 20 : 1 and 10 : 1 dilutions were mixed with 5 ml, 15 ml, and 30 ml of Hexabrix, which produced no response.

Another study by Mancini and McGillem compared Renografin 76 and Omnipaque (iohexol 300 mg/ml and 350 mg/ml) with two lots of the popular vasodilator papaverine HCl. One lot had a pH of 6.8 and the other had a pH of 7.2. The results indicated that Renografin 76 immediately formed a white suspension, and it formed a precipitate at 15 minutes and 12 hours when mixed with the 6.8-pH papaverine HCl. With the 7.2-pH papaverine HCl, Renografin 76 formed no immediate suspension, but a precipitate was noted at 12 hours. The two Omnipaque contrast medium agents did not demonstrate a response with either papaverine HCl lot. Mancini and McGillem's study was performed after they read the results of Pilla and coworkers. Pilla and associates became aware of the Mancini and McGillem's test results and attribute the differences between the two studies to the higher pH value used by Mancini and McGillem.

The above studies were performed *in vitro* (outside the human body). Shah and Gerlock reported an *in vivo* (within the human body) case study with Hexabrix and papaverine HCl. In this case report, three angiograms were performed on the same patient during the same catheterization period. The first was an aortogram using MD-76 (diatrizoate meglumine sodium). The second angiogram was a bilateral aortofemoral runoff study using Hexabrix mixed with 50 mg of 1% lidocaine. In both these studies, the patient's vessels remained patent. In the third angiogram, 30 mg of papaverine HCl was mixed with 10 ml of normal saline and injected through the catheter. A second injection of Hexabrix was administered after the catheter was flushed with 10 ml of normal saline. Complete occlusion of the left common femoral artery was noted. A select angiogram of the left external iliac was performed with Hexabrix to assess the occlusion, and the vessel was found to be patent. Shah and Gerlock concluded that the 30 mg of papaverine HCl followed by Hexabrix caused the temporary occlusion. It should be noted that McGill and associates performed animal studies to duplicate, and try to explain, the findings of Shah and Gerlock. On the basis of their results, McGill and coworkers doubted that the occlusion reported by Shah and Gerlock was caused by an incompatibility of Hexabrix and papaverine HCl.

Because of their experience, Shah and Gerlock performed *in vitro* experiments of separate mixtures of Hexabrix with 30 mg of undiluted papaverine HCl, 30 mg of papaverine HCl diluted in 10 ml of normal saline, 150 mg of Tagamet (cimetidine hydrochloride), 0.5 ml of 1 : 1000 epinephrine, 10 units of Pitressin (vasopressin), 25 mg of Priscoline (tolazoline HCl), 100 μg of Tridil (nitroglycerin), 50 mg of lidocaine HCl, 1000 units of heparin sodium, and 50 mg of Benadryl (diphenhydramine HCl). There was no response when Hexabrix was mixed with epinephrine, Tridil, or lidocaine. Table 8–1 presents the results of the other combinations.

Irving and Burbridge mixed each of the following contrast media:

Hexabrix
Hypaque 60 (diatrizoate meglumine)
MD-60 (diatrizoate meglumine and diatrizoate sodium)
Omnipaque
Isovue (iopamidol)
Conray 60 (iothalamate meglumine)

with each of the following medications:

adrenalin (epinephrine HCl)
Benadryl
heparin
protamine (protamine sulfate)
papaverine HCl
ampicillin
Ilotycin (erythromycin glucceptate)
Garamycin (gentamicin sulfate)
Chloromycetin (chloramphenicol sodium succinate)
Tagamet
Solu-Cortef (hydrocortisone sodium succinate)
Solu-Medrol (methylprednisolone sodium succinate)

Of the combinations tested, when Benadryl, papaverine HCl, protamine, and Tagamet were mixed with Hexabrix, all demonstrated a precipitation that lasted at least 2 hours. A transient precipitation that cleared in less than 5 minutes formed when Garamycin and Hexabrix were mixed. Both an immediate precipitation, which cleared, and a 1 hour delayed precipitation formed with the Hypaque 60 and Benadryl mixture. A transient precipitation occurred with the papaverine

TABLE 8–1

**Results of Shah and Gerlock's *In Vitro* Experiments
Mixing Various Drugs with Hexabrix**

Pharmacological Agent	Result
Undiluted papaverine HCl	Dense, cloudy, white precipitate
Diluted papaverine HCl	Suspension with minimal precipitation that clears
Tolazoline HCl	Oily, then clears
Heparin sodium	Oily, then clears
Benadryl	Dense cloudy precipitate
Tagamet	Thread-like precipitates

HCl and Hypaque 60 mixture. Protamine and Hypaque 60 produced a persistent precipitation. Both immediate transient and delayed precipitation occurred when MD-60 was mixed with Benadryl and papaverine HCl, respectively (1 hour for Benadryl and 2 hours for papaverine HCl). There was a persistent precipitation when MD-60 was mixed with Protamine. All other contrast media and medication mixtures had no response. Table 8–2 is a summary of the experimental results of Irving and Burbridge.

Kim and coworkers performed *in vitro* studies comparing each of nine contrast media with 21 different medications. The nine contrast agents were Telebrix (ioxithalamate meglumine), Hypaque 50, Hypaque 60, Conray 60, Hexabrix 320, Ultravist (iopromide) 300, Ultravist 370, Iopamiro (iopamidol) 300, and Omnipaque 300. The following are the 21 medications used in the various experiments:

papaverine
Regitine (phentolamine mesylate)
Priscoline
Alprostadil (prostaglandin E_1)
Millisrol (nitroglycerin)
vasopressin
epinephrine 1 : 1000
Benadryl
cimetidine
Avil (pheniramine maleate)
penicillin G (benzylpenicillin sodium)

TABLE 8–2

Results of Irving and Burbridge's *In Vitro* Experiments

Drug	Omnipaque	Isovue	Hexabrix	MD-60	Hypaque 60	Conray 60
adrenalin	NR	NR	NR	NR	NR	NR
Benadryl	NR	NR	PP	TP, DP1	TP, DP1	NR
heparin	NR	NR	NR	NR	NR	NR
protamine	NR	NR	PP	PP	PP	NR
ampicillin	NR	NR	NR	NR	NR	NR
Ilotycin	NR	NR	NR	NR	NR	NR
Garamycin	NR	NR	NR	NR	NR	NR
Chloromycetin	NR	NR	NR	NR	NR	NR
Tagamet	NR	NR	PP	NR	NR	NR
Solu-Cortef	NR	NR	NR	NR	NR	NR
Solu-Medrol	NR	NR	NR	NR	NR	NR
papaverine HCl	NR	NR	PP	TP, DP2	TP	NR

NR = no response
PP = persistent precipitation (at least 2 hours)
TP = temporary precipitation that cleared within 5 minutes
DP1 = precipitation after 1 hour that persisted
DP2 = precipitation after 2 hours that persisted

ampicillin (ampicillin sodium)
Helocetin (chloramphenicol sodium succinate)
gentamicin
Valium (diazepam)
pethidine HCl (meperidine HCl)
lidocaine (lidocaine HCl)
heparin
protamine
urokinase
Whycort (hydrocortisone sodium succinate)

One milliliter of each medication was added to each of the nine contrast media.

Each mixture was shaken for 5 seconds and observed for any response immediately and at 1-minute and 30-minute intervals. Response categories were as follows: no response, temporary white suspension (dissipated <1 minute), persistent white suspension (persisted >1 minute), and precipitated after centrifugation. Table 8–3 summarizes the results of the experiments of Kim and associates.

From these research studies, the following can be concluded relative to mixing contrast media with other drugs:

1. Catheters and infusion tubes should be flushed with saline between injections of contrast medium and medications. This is especially true if Hexabrix is used following papaverine HCl.
2. Avoid using contrast medium to flush papaverine HCl.
3. To reduce the possibility of incompatibility of papaverine HCl and contrast media, for every 1 ml of papaverine HCl used, dilute it with 25 ml of normal saline.
4. Avoid administering Benadryl through a tube that was used for the injection of Hexabrix, MD-60, or Hypaque 60. Doing so may inactivate the Benadryl or occlude the tubing.
5. Avoid injecting Hexabrix through tubing being used to infuse Tagamet.
6. Flush the catheter with saline if Hexabrix, Hypaque 50, or Hypaque 60 is used with the vasodilator papaverine HCl, Regitine, or Priscoline.
7. Flush the catheter with saline if Hexabrix, Hypaque 50, or Hypaque 60 is used with the antihistamine Benadryl or cimetidine.
8. Flush the catheter with saline if Hexabrix, Hypaque 50, or Hypaque 60 is used with the sedative Valium, pethidine HCl, or protamine.

Besides the potential for incompatibility between contrast media and other medications injected through a common access device, incompatibility may result from a medication the patient is taking. Relative to imaging, the drug Glucophage, used for diabetes mellitus, is currently the primary medication that can result in adverse reaction if contrast medium is injected in the patient. The research conducted by Bristol-Myers Squibb Company, manufacturer of Glucophage, indicates that injecting contrast medium in a patient using Glucophage can cause

TABLE 8-3

Results of *In Vitro* Experiments of Kim and Associates

Drug	Telebrix	Hypaque 60	Hypaque 50	Conray 60	Hexabrix	Ultravist 300	Ultravist 370	Iopamidol	Omnipaque
papaverine HCl	NR	PC	TS	NR	PC	NR	NR	NR	NR
Regitine	NR	TS	TS	PC	PS	NR	NR	NR	NR
Priscoline	NR	NR	NR	NR	TS	NR	NR	NR	NR
Alprostadil	NR	NR	NR	NR	NR	NR	NR	NR	NR
Millisrol	NR	NR	NR	NR	NR	NR	NR	NR	NR
vasopressin	NR	NR	NR	NR	NR	NR	NR	NR	NR
epinephrine	NR	NR	NR	NR	NR	NR	NR	NR	NR
Benadryl	NR	PC	PC	NR	PC	NR	NR	NR	NR
cimetidine	NR	PS	NR	NR	PC	NR	NR	NR	NR
Avil	NR	NR	NR	NR	NR	NR	NR	NR	NR
penicillin	NR	NR	NR	NR	NR	NR	NR	NR	NR
ampicillin	NR	NR	NR	NR	NR	NR	NR	NR	NR
Helocetin	NR	NR	NR	NR	NR	NR	NR	NR	NR
gentamicin	NR	NR	NR	NR	PC	NR	NR	NR	NR
Valium	NR	PS	NR	NR	NR	NR	NR	NR	NR
pethidine HCl	NR	PC	PC	NR	NR	NR	NR	NR	NR
lidocaine	NR	NR	NR	NR	NR	NR	NR	NR	NR
heparin	NR	NR	NR	NR	NR	NR	NR	NR	NR
protamine	NR	PC	PC	NR	PC	NR	NR	NR	NR
urokinase	NR	NR	NR	NR	NR	NR	NR	NR	NR
Whycort	NR	NR	NR	NR	NR	NR	NR	NR	NR

NR = No response
TS = Temporary white suspension
PS = Persistent white suspension
PC = Persistent precipitation after centrifugation
Reprinted with permission from Kim, SH, Lee, HK, and Han, MC: Incompatibility of water soluble contrast media and intravascular pharmacologic agents: An in vitro study. Invest Radiol January 1992; 27(1):45.

TABLE 8–4

Diseases, Conditions, and Drugs That May Influence Thyroid Uptake Results

Disease/Condition	Contrast Medium	Drugs

Chronic liver disease
Iodide deficiency
Nephrosis
	Meglumine diatrizoate
	Oral cholecystography media
	Sodium diatrizoate
	Recovery from iodinated
	  contrast media
		Adrenal steroids
		Aminosalicylic acid
		Androgens
		Anticoagulants
		Antihistamines
		Benzodiazepines
		Cimetidine
		Clioquinol
		Corticotrophin
		Cytomel
		Diiodohydroxyquin (iodoquinol)
		Dilantin
		Epinephrine
		Expectorants (containing iodine)
		Fluorides
		Iodine tincture
		Lithium
		Lugol's solution
		Meprobamate
		Mineral supplements
		Morphine
		Perchlorates
		Phenylbutazone
		Propylthiouracil
		Rebound following suppression with
		  thyroid or antithyroid drugs
		Resorcinol
		SSKI
		Salicylates
		Sodium nitroprusside
		Sulfonamides
		Sulfonylureas
		Synthroid
		Tapazole
		Thiamazole
		Thiopental
		Thyroid extracts
		Thyrolar
		Thyroxine
		Tolbutamide
		Topical iodines
		Vitamin supplements

acute renal failure. Thus, it is recommended that Glucophage be withheld for at least 48 hours prior to and 48 hours subsequent to contrast medium injection. Glucophage therapy should not be reinstituted after contrast medium injection until it has been determined that the patient's renal function is normal.

FACTORS THAT MAY INFLUENCE RADIOPHARMACEUTICAL LOCALIZATION

Unlike contrast media, radiopharmaceuticals don't tend to cause adverse reactions that require intervention. The problems associated with radiopharmaceuticals are limited to the interference of disease or drugs with imaging results. Many drugs and diseases can influence the area in which radiopharmaceuticals localize. A drug or disease can cause the radiopharmaceutical to enter organs other than the target organ. This can result in a decrease in imaging known as a "cold spot." Conversely, a drug or disease may increase the normal concentration of the radiopharmaceutical in the target organ. This can result in an increase in imaging known as a "hot spot." In both instances, the drug or disease adversely affects the imaging results. Thus, it is important to know what diseases the patient has and the medications the patient is taking. Unfortunately, this information is not

TABLE 8–5

Diseases, Contrast Medium, and Drugs That May Influence Bone Imaging Results

Disease/Condition	Contrast Medium	Drugs
Carcinomas	Sodium diatrizoate	Aluminum carbonate
Diabetes mellitus		Aluminum
Hypercalcemia		Amphotericin B
Hyperthyroid		Calcitonin
Leukemia		Cimetidine
Sickle cell anemia		Cyclophosphamide
Urinary obstruction		Dialysate
		Doxorubicin
		Ferrous gluconate
		Ferrous sulfate
		Gentamicin
		Heparin
		Iron dextran
		Iron therapy (long term)
		Meperidine
		Phospho-Soda
		Potassium phosphate
		Steroid therapy (long term)
		Vincristine

always readily available. The following is a brief summary of factors that may influence the results of common radiopharmaceutical procedures.

Thyroid examinations assess the function of the thyroid. However, an excess of iodine in the body may interfere with the study. Several iodine-containing drugs are known to interfere with thyroid uptake. Also, some diseases may produce inaccurate thyroid uptake results. Table 8–4 is a list of common diseases or conditions and drugs that have been found to influence the results of thyroid imaging.

In bone imaging using radiopharmaceuticals, the ability to detect lesions is partially influenced by the ratio of radioactivity in the lesion to that in normal bone or soft tissues. Some drugs and disease states interfere with the transportation of the radiotracer to bone, reduce blood clearance of the radiopharmaceutical, or cause excessive localization of the tracer in other organs, which compromises the image. Table 8–5 is a list of common diseases, contrast medium, and drugs that have been found to influence bone images.

TABLE 8–6

Diseases, Conditions, and Drugs That May Influence Liver and Spleen Imaging Results

Disease/Condition	Drugs
Anemia	Acetaminophen
Atelectasis	Actinomycin
Biliary cirrhosis	Aluminum
Crohn's disease	Carmustine
Hemophilia	Chlorambucil
Infectious mononucleosis	Cyclophosphamide
Intra-abdominal abscess	Dextrose
Liver cirrhosis	Enflurane
Malignant melanoma	Epinephrine
Severe abdominal trauma	Ferrous gluconate
Trauma	Ferrous sulfate
	5-Fluorouracil
	Halothane
	Heparin
	Immunosuppressive agents
	Lomustine
	Magnesium sulfate
	Methotrexate
	Oxacillin
	Phenobarbital
	Steroid hormones
	Tetracycline
	Thyroid hormones
	Vincristine
	Vitamin B_{12}

Some drugs may produce inaccurate results when used during liver and spleen imaging. These drugs tend to produce changes in the amount of radioactivity localized in the liver and spleen. Common target organs of a change in uptake are the lungs, spleen, bone marrow, and kidneys. Table 8–6 is a summary of common diseases, conditions, and drugs that may influence liver and spleen imaging results.

Several drugs and some therapies can change the location of radiopharmaceuticals used for tumor and abscess assessment. Common examples are penicillins, diuretics, antineoplastic agents, and nonsteroidal anti-inflammatory drugs. These,

TABLE 8–7

Diseases, Conditions, Therapy, and Drugs That May Influence Tumor and Abscess Imaging Results

Disease/Condition/ Therapy	Drugs
Acute tubular necrosis	Adrenal steroids
Estrogen therapy	Aminoglycosides
Hyperprolactinemia	Amiodarone
Iron deficiency	Bleomycin
Leukemia	Calcium gluconate
Lymphoma	Cephalexin
Obesity	Cephalosporins
Pregnancy	Cisplatin
Renal failure	Clindamycin
	Cyclophosphamide
	Dialysate
	Diethylstilbestrol
	Digitalis
	Doxorubicin
	Furosemide
	Gentamicin
	Imipramine
	Iron dextran
	Methotrexate
	Nitrofurantoin
	Penicillin
	Phenobarbital
	Phenylbutazone
	Phenytoin
	Prednisone
	Reserpine
	Sulfonamides
	Thiazides
	Vincristine

TABLE 8-8

Diseases, Therapy, and Drugs That May Influence Hepatobiliary Imaging Results

Disease/Therapy	Drugs
Acute pancreatitis	Antimuscarinics
Alcoholism	Atropine
Fasting	Bethanechol
Hepatic artery chemotherapy	Cholecystokinin
Parenteral feeding	Exogenous hormones
	Meperidine
	Morphine
	Nicotinic acid
	Phenobarbital
	Sincalide

in addition to some other conditions or therapy, often shift the localization of the tracer to the lungs, breast, or thyroid. Table 8–7 summarizes common diseases, therapy, and drugs that may influence tumor and abscess imaging results.

Hepatobiliary imaging is another procedure in which the radiopharmaceutical's location can be altered by disease, producing inaccurate results. Table 8–8 summarizes some diseases, therapy, and drugs that may influence hepatobiliary imaging results.

TABLE 8-9

Diseases and Drugs That May Influence Myocardial Perfusion Imaging Results Using Thallium Chloride

Disease	Drugs
Chronic thyroiditis	Atenolol
Graves' disease	Dexamethasone
Hashimoto's disease	Digitalis
Hyperthyroidism	Dilantin
Masked primary hypothyroidism	Dipyridamole
Metastatic thyroid carcinoma	Furosemide
Plummer's disease	Isoproterenol
Simple goiter carcinoma	Isosorbide dinitrate
	Metoprolol
	Nadolol
	Phenytoin
	Propranolol
	Sodium bicarbonate

Several drugs can affect the localizing of thallium chloride, which is commonly used for myocardial studies. Table 8–9 lists common diseases and drugs that may influence myocardial perfusion imaging using thallium chloride.

BIBLIOGRAPHY

Fisher, HW: Incompatibilities between contrast media and pharmacologic agents [letter]. Radiology 162(3):875, 1987.

Irving, HD, and Burbridge, BE: Incompatibility of contrast agents with intravascular medications. Radiology 173(1):91, October 1989.

Kim, SH, Lee, HK, and Han, MC: Incompatibility of water soluble contrast media and intravascular pharmacologic agents: an in vitro study. Invest Radiol 27(1):45, January 1992.

Laven, DL, and Shaw, SM: Detection of drug interactions involving radiopharmaceuticals: a professional responsibility of the clinical pharmacist. J Pharm Pract 11(5):287, October 1989.

Mancini, GB, and McGillem, MJ: Papaverine as a coronary vasodilator [letter]. AJR 147:1095, November 1986.

McGill, JE, Rysavy, JA, and Frick, MD: Experimental investigations of the Hexabrix-papaverine interaction. Radiology 166(2):577, February 1988.

Pilla, TJ, Beshany, SE, and Shields, JB: Incompatibility of Hexabrix and papaverine. AJR 146(6):1300, June 1986.

Shah, SJ, and Gerlock, AJR: Incompatibility of Hexabrix and papaverine in peripheral arteriography. Radiology 162(3):619, March 1987.

Shaw, SM: Drugs and diseases that may alter the biodistribution or pharmacokinetics of radiopharmaceuticals. Pharm Int, p 293, December 1985.

Select Drug Administration Techniques

9

INTRODUCTION

As noted in Chapter 4, Pharmacology Overview, the four routes identified in this text for drugs to enter the body are enteral, parenteral, pulmonary, and topical. A variety of methods can be used to administer medication via the enteral and parenteral routes. Enteral medication may be administered by employing sublingual, buccal, oral, or rectal means. Parenteral administration of drugs includes intravenous, intra-arterial, intramuscular, intradermal, intrathecal, and subcutaneous injections. Most methods of administering drugs allow the patient to self-administer the medication, e.g., oral drugs, topical medications. This is especially true in the case of nonprescription or "over the counter" drugs. However, there are instances, especially in parenteral administration, when a qualified health care provider administers the medication.

This chapter addresses the most common methods of drug administration that a radiological sciences technologist is most apt to perform. These include the oral, intramuscular, and intravenous methods, each of which is discussed in depth. The reader is advised that numerous methods are used to administer drugs. Some, such as eye drops and inhalants, are rarely seen in an imaging department. Discussion of all the various types of drug administration is beyond the scope of this text.

PRECAUTIONS

Regardless of the method used to administer a drug, certain precautions should be taken. These include the five "rights":

- the right patient
- the right drug
- the right dose
- the right time
- the right route

It is also appropriate to note that the patient has a right to refuse medication. The technologist should never give medication to a patient who has refused to take the drug. Assuming there is patient consent and prior to administering any medication, it is essential that the correct drug be selected for the correct patient. The most reliable method to ensure that the correct patient is receiving the proper medication is to read the patient's name band. If the patient is an outpatient, it is possible that no name band was issued. In these cases, it is important to ask the patient his or her name. It is better to ask the question "What is your name?" rather than "Are you Mr. John Jones?"—the difference being that some patients, especially if medicated or elderly, may not be alert and will answer "yes" even if their name is not Mr. John Jones. Asking patients their name requires them to say their name. If you must go to the patient's room to give some preprocedural medication or contrast medium, do not assume the name on the bed is the same as that of the patient in the bed. The patient could be in the wrong bed. Again, it is best to read the patient's name band. When confirming the patient's name, read both the first and the last names. Some surnames (last names) are very similar to a person's first name. For example, some people have the name "John" as a surname. Also, the surname "Roberts" might be misunderstood for the first name "Robert."

To ensure that the correct drug is administered to the correct patient, it is recommended that the technologist check the name of the drug at least three times: when removing the drug container from its storage place, when removing the drug from its container (drawing up the drug), and before returning the container to its storage place, or in the case of single-dose containers, disposing of the container. It is recommended that the container be kept until the drug has been administered. Thus, if any reaction occurs, it is possible to reread the container to determine if the correct drug or dose was administered. Also, if an unusually large number of reactions are occurring, it is possible to check the control number of the drug to determine if there is a problem with that "batch" of medication.

Ensuring that the right dose is administered is as important as verifying that the correct patient is being given the correct drug. Care should be taken to read the container to determine the strength of the dose. For example, some parenteral drugs are sold in different strengths. Thus, it is possible to select the correct drug but the incorrect strength. Also, it is important for the technologist to be able to convert dose measurements. Thus, if the physician orders something in milliliters, but the drug container is in ounces, the technologist should know how to convert the dose (see Chapter 5, Drug Measurements and Dose Calculation).

Administration of some medication or contrast medium is time dependent. In other words, if contrast medium or sedation needs to be given 20–30 minutes prior to a computed tomography (CT) procedure, it is important that its administration to the patient be timely. Thus, the technologist needs to be aware of the time at which the patient will undergo the procedure prior to administering the medication. For example, if one patient's examination is delayed, causing the next patient's examination to start late, the administration of the medication to the next patient should be delayed to correspond with the correct preprocedural time for administering the medication.

Some medications may be administered using different routes. It is important that the technologist confirm the route ordered by the physician prior to administering the medication.

Besides the five "right" rules, the technologist should follow other precautions. These include periodically rereading the insert that comes with the drug. Thousands of drugs are on the market, and new ones evolve regularly. Also, it is possible that the method of administering the drug, indications, contraindications, etc., may change as more is learned about the drug. Thus, it is important to refresh one's memory regarding the information about the medication.

Another precaution the technologist should adhere to is to question any order that is unclear or unusual. For example, if the physician orders a dose of a drug that is routinely given at a lower dose, the technologist should repeat the order and ask the doctor if he or she wishes to administer the higher dose.

When preparing or administering drugs, technologists should direct their undivided attention to the task at hand. Talking to someone while preparing or administering medication should be avoided because it distracts from the task at hand.

It is important for the technologist to stay with the patient during and after the administration of the medication. This means that the technologist should not hand a patient contrast medium to drink and then leave before the patient has completely ingested the liquid. The patient might not drink the medication or may aspirate while drinking it. Thus, the technologist should be present to handle any unforeseen events due to the administration of the medication.

Besides the above "right" rules and precautions, some "don'ts" are associated with the administration of drugs. These include:

1. Don't use a drug without a label on it or if the label is illegible.
2. Don't give a drug to a patient that was prepared by someone else.
3. Don't chart or record a medication as given until the patient has actually taken the drug.

ORAL ADMINISTRATION OF DRUGS

The oral route is the simplest and safest method for drug administration. Oral medications are packaged in a variety of forms. These include, but are not limited to, capsules, emulsions, lozenges, suspensions, syrups, granules, and tablets. In an imaging department, the most common form of oral medication is suspension although sometimes a tablet, granule, capsule, or pill may be given. In this text, the discussion of oral administration of drugs is limited to the types of medications most apt to be utilized in an imaging department.

ADMINISTRATION OF PILLS

All methods of drug administration require use of aseptic technique. Thus, prior to any drug administration, it is important for technologists to wash their hands.

After the technologist washes his or her hands according to facility protocol, the drug to be administered is selected, using the precautions noted in the pre viously discussed "right" rules. A clean souffle cup (medicine cup) is also obtained. For preparation of the correct dose, the medication container and souffle cup are placed on a clean surface that is clear of other items.

To prepare the correct dose, grasp the medication container (checking to make sure you have the correct medication) with your dominant hand and open it (unscrew the lid) using your nondominant hand (Fig. 9–1A). Remove the lid and turn it upside-down. Without touching the medication, shake or tap the container so that the appropriate quantity of medication falls into the lid of the container (see Fig. 9–1B). Place the opened container in a safe place on the counter and put the lid, with the medication, in your dominant hand. Hold the souffle cup with your nondominant hand and, without touching the drug, pour

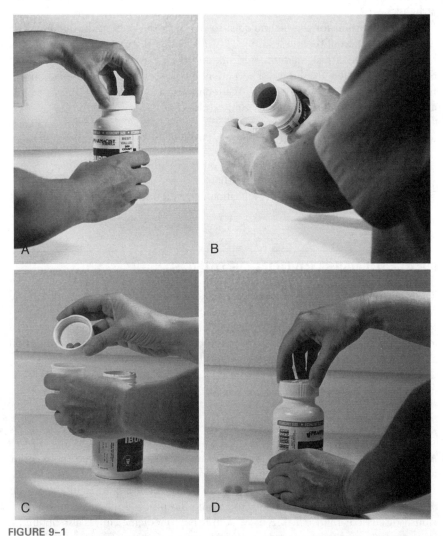

FIGURE 9–1
Preparing the correct oral dose of a solid drug. A. Open the container. B. Turn the lid upside-down and shake the container until the appropriate quantity of the drug is in the lid of the container. If the container is being used for the first time, there may be a need to remove a protective seal. C. Pour the drug into the souffle cup. D. Replace the lid on the open container.

the medication from the lid into the souffle cup (see Fig. 9–1*C*). Place the souffle cup, with the medication, in a safe place on the counter and hold the open container with your nondominant hand. Replace the cap on the open container (see Fig. 9–1*D*). Again, check the name of the medication to ensure that it is correct and return the container to its proper storage place.

Obtain a glass of water for the patient to drink during drug administration. Pick up the souffle cup and glass of water and walk to the patient. Verify the patient's name as indicated in the "right" rules. Explain what you are doing and what the medication is used for. Answer any questions the patient may ask about the medication or procedure. Make sure the patient is in an upright position and instruct the patient on how to take the medication. Advise the patient to take a small sip of the water and to then take the medication with additional water. Hand the souffle cup and glass of water to the patient. Stay with the patient until he or she has taken it. Take the empty water and souffle cups from the patient. Properly dispose of the cups and wash your hands. Note in the chart the medication you administered (see Chapter 10, Documentation, for proper charting methods).

Sometimes patients have difficulty swallowing oral medication. It is possible to facilitate swallowing medication by instructing the patient to drink before taking the drug. It is recommended that the patient not lean the head backward because this tends to increase the possibility of choking. Rather, the patient should lean forward while taking the medication. Also, massaging the laryngeal prominence (Adam's apple) or just under the chin sometimes assists in swallowing. To ensure that the medication is in the stomach, it is recommended that the patient drink at least 3 oz of water. The water also serves to decrease the risk of the medication irritating the gastrointestinal tract.

ADMINISTRATION OF LIQUIDS

As with all drug administration, prior to administering liquid medication, it is important for technologists to wash their hands. After hand washing, the drug to be administered is selected using the precautions previously discussed for the "right" rules. A cup that the medication will be poured into is also obtained.

Many liquid medications need to be thoroughly mixed (shaken) before being given to the patient. Thus, the technologist should read the label and shake the container, if appropriate, prior to pouring the medication into a cup.

To pour the medication into a cup, open the lid of the container and place it upside-down in a safe clean spot on the counter (Fig. 9–2*A*). Placing the lid upside-down will help prevent contamination of the lid. Grasp the container in your dominant hand with the label facing upward, toward the ceiling (see Fig. 9–2*B*). This will prevent the liquid from accidentally dripping on the label and possibly obscuring it. Containers whose handles are opposite the label (e.g., some large barium containers) make it difficult to pour the liquid with the label facing upward. Hold the cup with your nondominant hand and pour the appropriate dose into the cup. When the appropriate amount of medication has been reached,

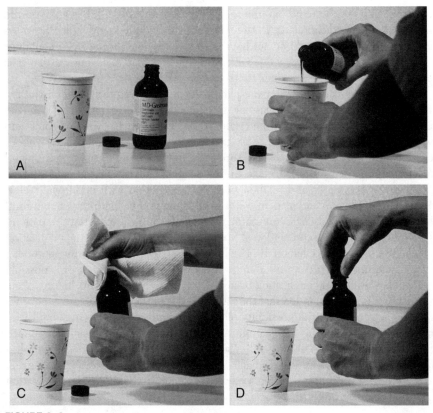

FIGURE 9–2
Preparing the correct oral dose of a liquid drug. *A.* Open the container, placing the lid upside down on the counter. *B.* While holding the container with the label facing upward, pour the liquid into the glass. *C.* Wipe the container. *D.* Recap the container.

place the cup and container in a safe place on the counter. Wipe off any excess liquid that may have dripped on the container (see Fig. 9–2*C*), recap the container (see Fig. 9–2*D*), and return it to its storage place or dispose of it properly (again, rechecking the name of the drug to ensure that it is correct). It should be noted that some liquid medication, e.g., contrast media, may contain more medication than can be held in a cup. Thus, the cup must be refilled. Also, when the medication needs to be measured, it should be poured in a clear, see-through cup held at eye level to ensure the proper dose.

Pick up the medication and walk to the patient. Verify the patient's name as indicated in the "right" rules. Explain what you are doing and what the medication is used for. Answer any questions the patient may ask about the medication or procedure. Make sure the patient is in an upright position and instruct the patient on how to take the medication. Hand the medication to the patient. Stay with the patient until he or she has drunk all the medication. Take the empty cup from the patient. Properly dispose of the cup and wash your hands. Note in the chart the medication that you administered (see Chapter 10, Documentation, for proper charting methods).

ADMINISTRATION OF LIQUIDS THROUGH A NASOGASTRIC TUBE

Sometimes patients are unable to swallow and have a nasogastric (NG) tube. This tube is placed in the nose and passes through the esophagus into the stomach (Fig. 9–3). The portion of the tube that is outside the patient has a clamp on it to prevent the back flow of liquid.

It may become necessary to administer medication through the NG tube. When medication is administered through the NG tube, it bypasses the normal digestive process undergone in the mouth (with saliva) and esophagus (with esophageal juices). Most medications administered in an imaging department through a NG tube are liquids. A syringe and tapered adaptor are needed to inject the medication into the tube.

Attach the tapered adaptor to the tubing (Fig. 9–4A). Attach a sterile syringe to the opposite end of the adaptor (see Fig. 9–4B). Withdraw the plunger of the syringe (see Fig. 9–4C). This checks the placement of the NG tube to ensure that it is located in the stomach. If it is in the stomach, stomach fluid should flow back. If no fluid is seen, 5–10 ml of air may be injected into the tube while a stethoscope is placed over the stomach. If a gurgling sound is heard in the stomach when the air is injected, the tube is positioned correctly. After verifying that the tube is positioned correctly, clamp the tube and remove the syringe (see Fig.

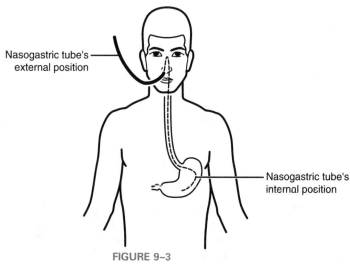

Nasogastric tube's external position

Nasogastric tube's internal position

FIGURE 9–3
Position of nasogastric tube.

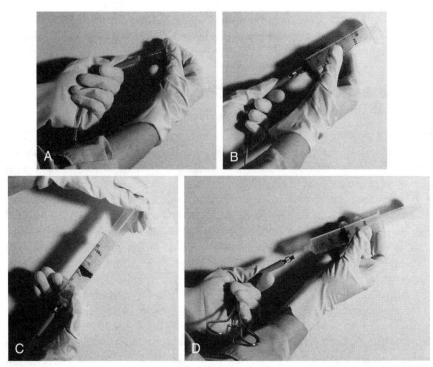

FIGURE 9–4

Injecting medication through a Levin nasogastric (NG) tube. *A.* Attach tapered adaptor to the NG tube. *B.* Attach a syringe to the adaptor. *C.* Withdraw the plunger of the syringe to verify the location of the tube. *D.* Clamp the tube and remove the syringe.

Illustration continued on opposite page

9–4*D*). Remove the plunger of the syringe and reattach the barrel of the syringe to the tube (see Fig. 9–4*E*). Hold the syringe above the patient and at a 90-degree angle to the ground. Unclamp the tubing and slowly pour the medication into the barrel of the syringe (see Fig. 9–4*F*). The force of gravity will allow the medication to flow into the stomach. After the medication has been administered, flush the tube with 15–50 ml (the amount is determined by the size of the tube) of water. Remove the tapered adaptor and barrel of the syringe and reclamp the tubing (see Fig. 9–4*G*).

FUNDAMENTALS OF PARENTERAL INJECTIONS

Parenteral drug administration uses methods other than those used in the enteral, pulmonary, or topical routes. These include the intravenous, intra-arterial, intramuscular, intradermal, intrathecal, and subcutaneous methods. Regardless of which route is used for injection, technologists should adhere to common fundamental care protocols when performing a parenteral injection. These deal with

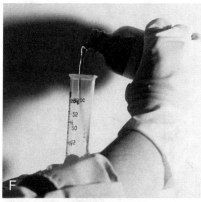

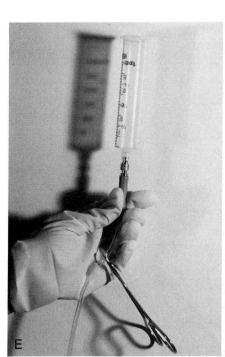

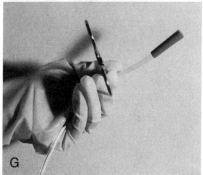

FIGURE 9-4 (*Continued*)

E. Remove the plunger of the syringe and reattach the barrel of the syringe to the tube. *F.* Unclamp the tube and pour the medication into the barrel of the syringe. *G.* Remove the tapered adaptor and barrel of the syringe and reclamp the tubing.

the drawing up of the medication. Prior to providing specific information on the correct method of drawing up medication for parenteral injection, a discussion on syringes, needles, and types of drug containers is in order.

A syringe and needle are required to draw up medication for parenteral injection. Many types of syringes are commercially available (Fig. 9-5). These include tuberculin, insulin, and standard syringes and reusable medication cartridge holder. The tuberculin syringe holds a maximum of 1 ml of medication. Insulin syringes are graduated in units rather than cubic centimeters or milliliters. The standard syringe is available in 3, 5, 10, 20, 25, 30, 35, and 50 ml sizes. The reusable medication cartridge holder must be used with a prefilled cartridge that contains the medication to be injected. It is important to select the correct syringe when performing parenteral injections.

Syringes can be disassembled. The parts of a syringe include the barrel, plunger, and tip (Fig. 9-6). Syringes may be made of plastic (disposable) or glass (reusable). Although the majority of syringes used are plastic, sometimes glass syringes must be used for medications that are incompatible with plastic.

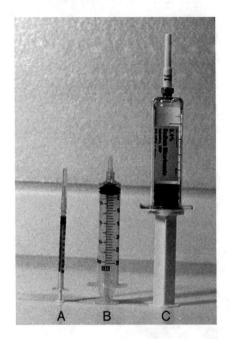

FIGURE 9-5
Types of syringes. *A.* Tuberculin. *B.* Standard (available in 3, 5, 10, 20, 25, 30, 35, and 50 ml sizes). *C.* Medication cartridge holder.

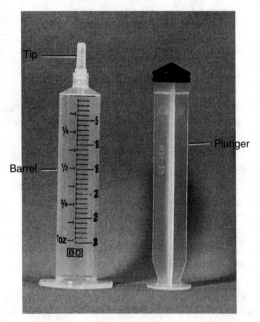

FIGURE 9-6
Syringe parts.

Needles, like syringes, also come in a variety of types (Fig. 9–7). Common needle types include the scalp vein (butterfly), intracatheter (angiocath), and standard hypodermic needles. The scalp vein needle has small thin tubing attached to the hub of the needle. It also has plastic "wings" on the sides that can be pinched to assist in needle insertion. The intracatheter has a metal needle located inside a soft plastic tube, or catheter. The needle projects out the end of the catheter and is used to puncture the skin. After the needle is properly placed in a vein, the needle is removed, leaving only the catheter in the vessel.

Needles consist of a hub, shaft, and bevel (Fig. 9–8). The hub is used to attach items such as a syringe. The bevel is angled and sharp. It is used to perform the puncture. The longer the bevel, the easier the puncture. The shaft varies in length from ½ inch to 3 inches. The diameter of the needle is measured in a unit called gauge. The larger the gauge number, the smaller the diameter of the needle.

It is important to select the proper needle and syringe for parenteral injection. The factors involved in determining the type of syringe and needle to use include the location of the injection site, the size of the patient, the type of medication being injected, and the age of the patient. Smaller syringes are used for small doses. Short needle lengths are used for intradermal injections, on children, and with elderly patients who have some muscle atrophy. The longer needles are used when there is a need to puncture deeper or on larger patients and to prevent a "whipping" effect of the cannula during rapid bolus injection. Small-gauge, large-lumen needles, e.g., 18-gauge, are used for thick liquid solutions such as blood. Larger gauges are used for thin liquid solutions.

The medication used for parenteral injection is stored in a vial, mix-o-vial, prefilled tube or cartridge, or ampule (Fig. 9–9). A vial usually contains multiple doses. It has a rubber stopper with an aluminum cover. To draw up the medication, the aluminum cover is removed and the top is cleaned with alcohol (the top does

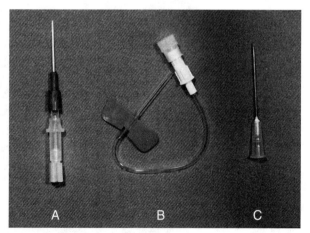

FIGURE 9–7
Types of needles. *A.* Intracatheter. *B.* Butterfly. *C.* Standard hypodermic.

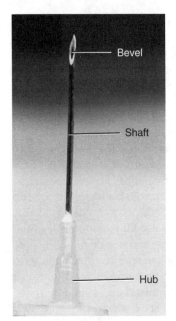

FIGURE 9–8
Needle parts.

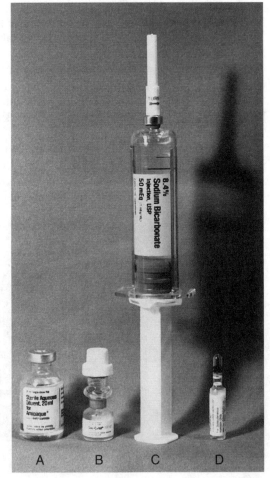

FIGURE 9–9
Medication containers. *A.* Vial. *B.*
Dual-compartment mix-o-vial. *C.*
Prefilled tubes. *D.* Ampule.

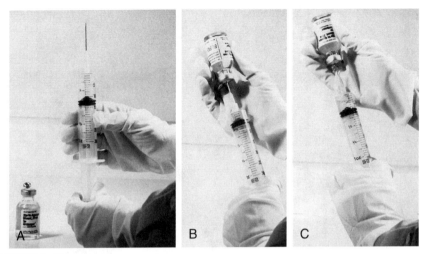

FIGURE 9-10
Filling a syringe from a vial. *A.* Open the vial and withdraw the barrel of the syringe to the amount of ml to be drawn up. *B.* Insert the barrel into the syringe and inject air into the vial. *C.* The medication flows into the barrel of the syringe.

not have to be cleaned if being used for the first time). The plunger of the syringe is withdrawn to the quantity of dose desired. The needle is inserted into the vial, bevel up, and the plunger is inserted in the syringe, injecting air into the vial. The pressure difference between the vial and syringe results in the medication's filling the barrel of the syringe. Make sure the tip of the needle is always in the solution. Figure 9–10 demonstrates how to fill a syringe from a vial. A mix-o-vial is designed so that the user injects sterile water or saline into the glass vial containing the powdered medication, or it may have two separate compartments, one containing the sterile solution and the other containing the powdered medication. If the mix-o-vial requires the user to inject sterile water or saline, the technologist must draw up the appropriate quantity of sterile solution, clean the top of the vial, and inject the solution (Fig. 9–11). In the dual-compartment vial, the user pushes the stopper down, which opens the compartment separator, allowing the solution and powder to mix (Fig. 9–12). In both cases, the user should roll the vial, i.e., between the hands, to mix (reconstitute) the medication. Do not shake the vial to reconstitute the solution. Prefilled tubes or cartridges contain a single dose and are designed to be used quickly, e.g., in case of cardiac arrest. Use of a prefilled tube requires a cartridge holder (Fig. 9-13) Ampules are single-dose glass medicine containers. They have a long, thin top that is weakened at the neck by the manufacturer to facilitate opening it. To open an ampule, wrap the neck of the ampule with a piece of gauze around the weakened area of the neck, curling the fingers of one hand around the body of the ampule and the fingers of the other hand around the top of the ampule. Place the thumbs

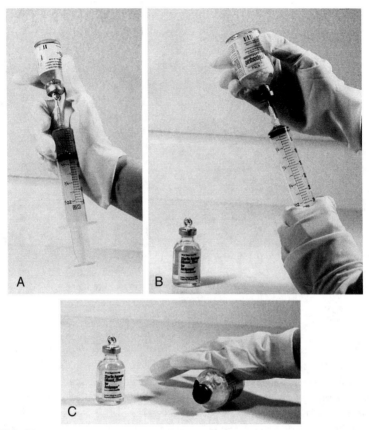

FIGURE 9–11
To mix the powdered medication with sterile water or saline: *A.* Draw up the appropriate quantity of sterile solution. *B.* Inject the sterile solution into the vial. *C.* Roll the vial to mix the medication.

of each hand on the gauze and over the neck of the ampule (Fig. 9–14*A*). The neck of the ampule is then broken by applying pressure on the weakened portion in a direction away from the body (see Fig. 9–14*B*). Insert the plunger of the syringe into the barrel of the syringe. Put a needle on the syringe. Tip the ampule so that the drug is near the top and place the needle of the syringe into the ampule. Pull back on the plunger to withdraw the medication (see Fig. 9–14*C*). Make sure the medication always covers the end of the needle. This may require increasing the tilt of the ampule. Care should be taken to prevent cutting oneself or allowing small pieces of glass to fall into the ampule. Filtered needles can be purchased to withdraw the medication. The filtered needle allows the liquid to pass through to the syringe, but will not allow any glass particles to enter the syringe. The needle used to withdraw the medication should be disposed of, and a new needle should be attached to the syringe for injection.

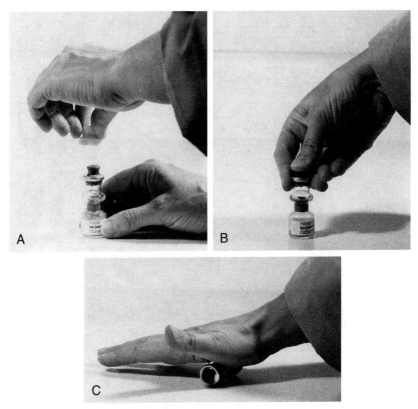

FIGURE 9-12
To use a dual-compartment vial: *A.* Open the top. *B.* Push down on the rubber stopper. *C.* Roll the vial to mix the medication.

INTRAMUSCULAR INJECTION

INTRAMUSCULAR INJECTION SITES

The most common type of parenteral administration is the intramuscular approach. As the name implies, the intramuscular approach is the injection of medication into a muscle. The quantity of medication injected at any one site using the intramuscular approach ranges from 1 ml to 5 ml. If 5 ml is the dose, two injections of 2.5 ml at different locations should be given to reduce pain. Sites for intramuscular injection are the deltoid, ventrogluteal, dorsogluteal, vastus lateralis, and rectus femoris muscles (Fig. 9–15). These sites are desirable because they contain few nerves or blood vessels. The deltoid, ventrogluteal, and dorsogluteal sites are not recommended for children because the muscles in these areas are not developed yet. The deltoid site is not used often because it has a higher blood flow than other sites and is able to accommodate only 2 ml of medication

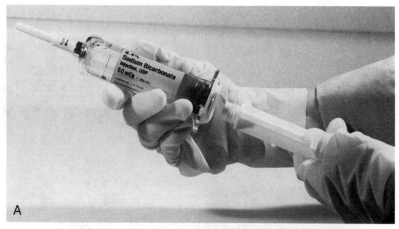

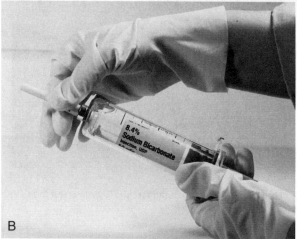

FIGURE 9–13
To use a prefilled cartridge: *A.* Thread the plastic rod into the plunger tip, which is located inside the barrel of the syringe. *B.* Turn the needle guard in the direction of the arrow located on the guard.

or less. The site should be rotated when performing multiple injections. Avoid injecting in areas that are bruised, scarred, or swollen from previous injections.

Deltoid injections should occur in the mid-deltoid area (see Fig. 9–15A). The patient is either upright or supine for the injection. The site of injection can be located by drawing an invisible line across the lowest (inferior) edge of the acromion. Imaginary lines are drawn from each end of the acromion (perpendicular) line downward to the midpoint of the axillary. The desired point of injection is in the middle of this imaginary rectangle.

In the ventrogluteal injection, the patient is supine with the toes pointed inward to relax the muscle or lying on his or her side. To locate the site, place

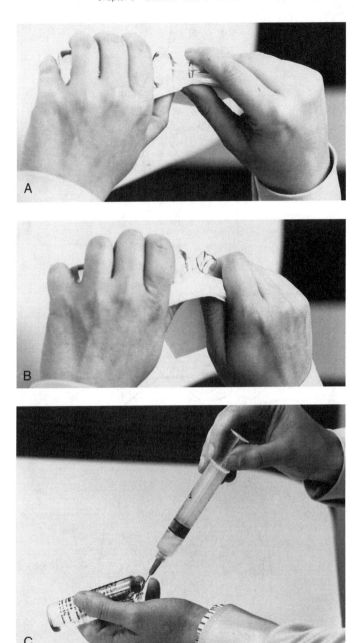

FIGURE 9–14
Withdrawal of medication from an ampule. *A.* Grasp the weakened area of the neck of the ampule with gauze. *B.* Break the neck of the ampule (away from the body). *C.* Withdraw the medication. (Courtesy of Tortorici, MR, and Apfel, PJ: Advanced radiographic and angiographic procedures with an introduction to specialized imaging. F. A. Davis, Philadelphia, 1995.)

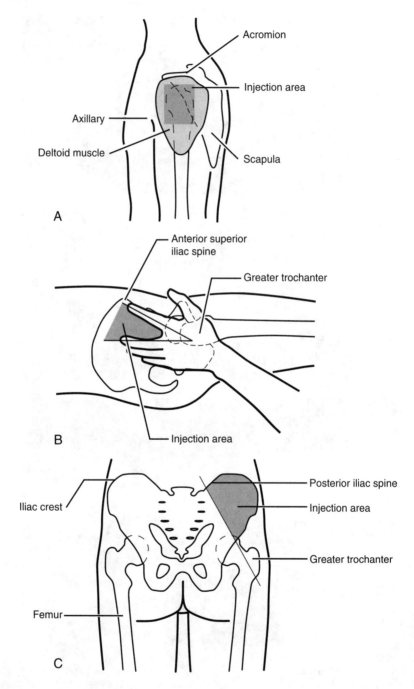

FIGURE 9–15
Intramuscular injection sites. *A.* Deltoid (patient is erect). *B.* Ventrogluteal (patient is supine). *C.* Dorsogluteal (patient is prone).

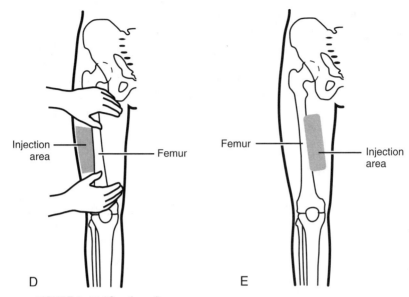

FIGURE 9–15 (*Continued*)
D. Vastus lateralis (patient is supine). *E.* Rectus femoris (patient is supine).

the palm of the hand opposite the side of injection (if injecting the right side, use the left hand) on the greater trochanter. Point the index finger to the anterior superior iliac spine and middle figure toward the iliac crest (see Fig. 9–15*B*). Inject in the center of the V shape formed by the fingers.

For a dorsogluteal injection, the patient is prone with the toes pointed inward to relax the muscle. An imaginary line is drawn from the greater trochanter to the posterior iliac spine (see Fig. 9–15*C*). The injection should be below the imaginary line and inferior to the iliac crest.

The vastus lateralis site is most commonly used for children because it is more developed than the other locations. Place the patient supine to locate the injection site, which is on the upper outer part of the leg one hand width below the greater trochanter and one hand above the knee (see Fig. 9–15*D*).

The rectus femoris muscle is useful in self-injections because it is easily located. It is also used for children. The muscle is located on the anterior portion of the thigh and at the level of the midshaft of the femur (see Fig. 9–15*E*). The muscle is medial to the vastus lateralis and does not extend beyond the midline of the anterior portion of the thigh. Care should be taken if using this site because it contains many blood vessels and is close to the sciatic nerve.

INTRAMUSCULAR INJECTION TECHNIQUE

Prior to performing an intramuscular injection, the technologist should follow the usual "right" rules, precautions, and preparation. After the technologist has performed the proper preprocedural care, the injection site is exposed and cleaned using alcohol, an iodine antiseptic solution, or both to clean the site. Iodine solutions should be avoided if the patient is allergic to iodine and for an intradermal injection in which the skin has to be visualized. To clean the skin, start at the center of the injection site and use circular motions moving outward from the center for about 2 inches. Allow time for the solution to dry. Do not blow (or fan) the site to dry it or inject while the solution is still wet because this increases the possibility of infection.

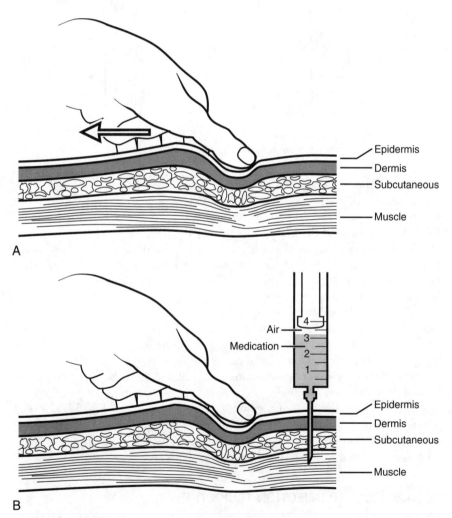

FIGURE 9-16
Z-track injection method. A. Pull the skin laterally. B. Insert the needle at 90 degrees.

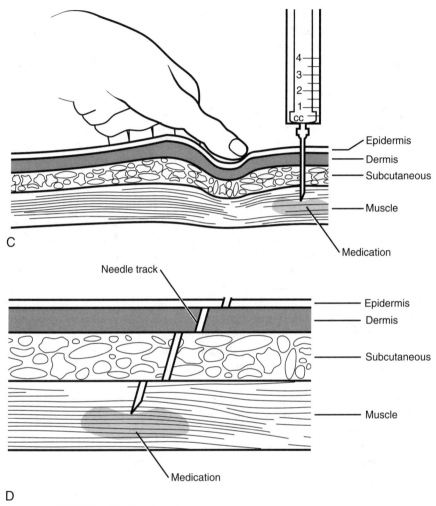

FIGURE 9–16 (*Continued*)
C. Inject the medication. *D.* Remove the needle and release the skin.

To insert the needle, hold the syringe like a dart with your dominant hand. Use the index finger and thumb of your nondominant hand to stretch the skin taut. Position the needle so that it makes a 90-degree angle with the skin and is about 2 inches from the injection site. Using a quick jab, insert three fourths of the needle in the injection site so that the needle enters the muscle. With the nondominant hand, securely hold the syringe. To make sure the needle is in the muscle and not a vessel, use the dominant hand to withdraw the plunger. If a red color appears, it means the needle is in a vessel. In this case, withdraw the needle and reinject in another location using a new needle, syringe, and medication. When the needle is in the proper position, inject the medication. After injecting the medication, record the appropriate information in the patient's chart (see Chapter 10, Documentation, for more information).

To withdraw the needle, use a clean gauze or cotton pad and withdraw the needle. Apply firm pressure to the puncture site. You may massage the site as long as the medication used does not prohibit the muscle from being massaged, as is the case with heparin. Properly dispose of the needle and syringe. Place a bandage on the injection site to prevent bleeding.

If the medication is irritating or a permanent stain may occur in the superficial tissues, a Z-track method of injection may be used (Fig. 9–16). The dorsogluteal muscle is usually used because of its large size. In this method, the routine procedure is used to draw up the medication, with the addition of drawing up 0.2–0.5 ml of air. The air ensures that no medication is left in the needle, helps seal the needle track, and prevents any back flow of the medication through the needle "track." The needle used to draw up the medication is replaced with a new needle. This will prevent any irritating medication that might be in the needle from coming in contact with the tissue. The nondominant hand pulls the skin laterally. The needle is inserted at a 90-degree angle to the skin, and the position is verified by withdrawing the plunger to check whether blood returns. Inject the medication slowly and wait 5–10 seconds to prevent the medication from seeping into the needle track. Remove the needle and release the skin. This will seal the needle track. Do not massage the area or allow the patient to wear tight clothing over the site because this may cause the medication to enter the subcutaneous tissue, resulting in irritation. Absorption of the medication may be increased by muscle activity such as walking.

Most pain associated with intramuscular injections is a result of several factors. These include stretching of the skin, the drug itself, the diameter of the needle (the larger the diameter, the more pain), unsteady injection, aspiration, site used (the thinner the tissue at the site, the more nerves, the more possibility of pain), and displacement or compression of the tissue caused by the volume (space) occupied by the drug. A dose larger than 1.5–2.5 ml should be administered in two injections at different locations to decrease the volume and subsequent pain.

INTRAVENOUS INJECTION

Intravenous (IV) injection is performed when large doses of medication need to be given, in cases of emergency, or if a medication cannot be administered by any other means. As the name indicates, IV injections involve the administering of a drug into a vein. Because the medication is injected in the blood stream, its effect is almost immediate. Also, it is impossible to remove a drug once it has been injected. Thus, care needs to be taken to verify the drug, dose, patient, route, and time.

Many hospitals have an IV team that is responsible for starting, troubleshooting, and removing IV lines. It is not uncommon for the technologist to perform venipuncture and inject even in institutions having IV teams.

A variety of IV methods are used to administer medication. These include a direct bolus injection, continuous infusion, adding medication to an IV bag, adding medication to a volume control chamber, and adding medication through the IV line. The most common types of injections in an imaging department are the direct injection, i.e., of radioisotopes, the continuous infusion method, i.e., of contrast media for IV pyelography, and adding medication through the IV line. Thus, the following discussion is limited to these areas.

Because this text is designed for the registered technologist or student completing his or her education, it is assumed that the reader has the experience and knowledge to properly change or assist in establishing an IV bottle or bag, knows how to regulate the medication flow, and can use an infusion pump.

FUNDAMENTALS OF INTRAVENOUS INJECTION

As indicated previously, a variety of needles and syringes can be used for parenteral injection. The equipment used for IV injection depends on the puncture site chosen, type of injection, and degree of irritation of the medication. If the puncture site has small vessels, then a large-gauge needle (one of small diameter) should be employed. For a bolus injection, selection of a large vessel with use of a small-gauge needle is recommended. Medications that are irritating should be delivered in large vessels with large-gauge needles. This increases the dilution of the drug in the blood and helps reduce irritation.

The most common sites for IV injection are in the forearm, wrist, and hand. The veins most often punctured in the hand and wrist are the dorsal metacarpal, cephalic, and basilic veins (Fig. 9–17A). The most common sites in the forearm are the ventral veins of the elbow and basilic, cephalic, and median cubital veins (see Fig. 9–17B). Other less popular sites are the superficial veins in the leg and foot. However, use of these veins is discouraged because puncturing them increases the potential for phlebitis. The subclavian, internal jugular, and external jugular veins are used for long-term therapy. A scalp vein is a common site of injection for infants and small children.

IV administration is similar to intramuscular administration of drugs in that prior to performing the injection, the usual "right" rules, precautions, and preparation are followed. After the technologist performs the proper preprocedural care, the injection site is exposed and assessed to determine the status of the veins. Veins, unlike muscles, present unique problems. The potential difficulties include deep location of veins (as often seen with obese patients), friable vessels (seen in debilitated or elderly patients), movable veins (as often seen with elderly patients), and tortuous vessels. Assessment involves visually inspecting and palpating the vein area. Besides the specific puncture site, it is important to assess the overall physical health of the patient. For example, if a patient has undergone a unilateral

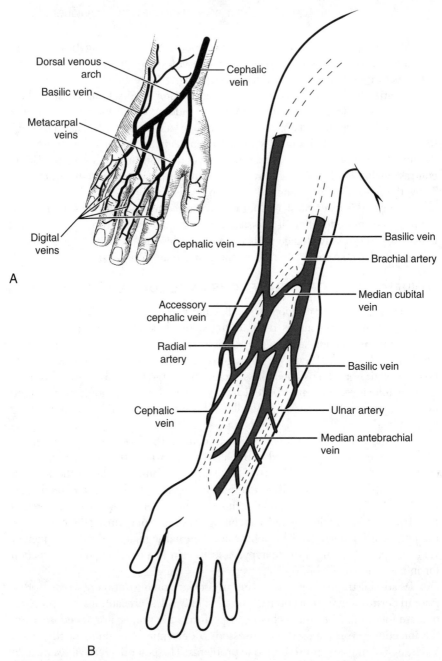

FIGURE 9–17
Common intravenous injection sites. *A.* The hand and wrist. (Reprinted with permission from Shila, RC: Manual for therapy procedures. 2nd ed. PMIC, Los Angeles, 1985.) *B.* The forearm. (Reprinted with permission from Plumer, AC: Principles and practices of intravenous therapy, 3rd ed. Little, Brown, Boston, 1982.)

mastectomy or has a fistula or shunt, the puncture should be made on the side opposite these conditions. After the site has been located, the area is cleansed.

The cleansing of the puncture site is similar to that for intramuscular technique, the primary difference being in the solutions used to clean the skin. Because visualization of the vein is important, if an iodine antiseptic solution is used to clean the site, an alcohol swab should be used to reclean the area. This helps remove the dark staining caused by the iodine, which may obscure visualization of the vein.

Besides selecting the appropriate needle, the other equipment needed for a venipuncture includes a tourniquet, alcohol swabs or an iodophor (iodine) solution, 2″ × 2″ gauze, cotton pad, paper or silk tape, and a bedsaver. The tourniquet is used to block the venous flow of blood while maintaining the arterial flow. A tourniquet should be attached to the patient about 6–10 inches proximal to the puncture site and using a slip knot (Fig. 9–18). A wide (at least 1 inch in diameter) tourniquet is recommended for children and elderly patients because it decreases discomfort. Also, the use of a gently inflated blood pressure cuff (to about diastolic pressure level) on children and patients with friable vessels helps decrease discomfort and minimize the trauma to the vessel. The alcohol swabs, iodophor solution, and cotton pad are used to clean the skin. The gauze is used to apply pressure to the puncture site. Tape is used to secure the needle and label the time and date of the puncture. To protect the table or bed from being soiled, a bedsaver is employed.

Proper puncture requires the vein to be distended. The tourniquet is used to dilate the vein. However, the tourniquet may not always distend the vein to a point of facilitating the puncture. Several techniques may be used to help increase the dilation of the vein. These include having the patient open and close his or her hand, placing the hand below the heart level, milking the vessel (massaging the vessel from the proximal to distal end), using a blood pressure cuff inflated to slightly above diastolic pressure, using hot compression (about 105° F), and gently tapping the puncture site. It should be noted that research performed by Don and colleagues indicated that slapping the vein may increase the potassium concentration in the blood. Thus, if the patient is to undergo blood work in which the potassium content is assessed, the test may give a false-positive reading if the patient's vein was slapped during venipuncture just prior to the blood test.

There are two types of punctures, direct and indirect (Fig. 9–19). The direct method is recommended for patients with tough skin, whereas the indirect method is useful in patients with fragile or rolling veins. In the direct method, the skin is cleansed, and a tourniquet is applied. The thumb of the nondominant hand pulls the skin taut. Using the dominant hand, the needle is placed, bevel up, at about a 45-degree angle to the skin, about ½ inch below the puncture site and directly over the vein. With a constant smooth "push," the needle is inserted. The angle of the needle is reduced (almost parallel to the skin), and the needle is advanced slightly in the vein. Location is verified by withdrawing the plunger to obtain a blood back flow. The difference between the direct and indirect methods

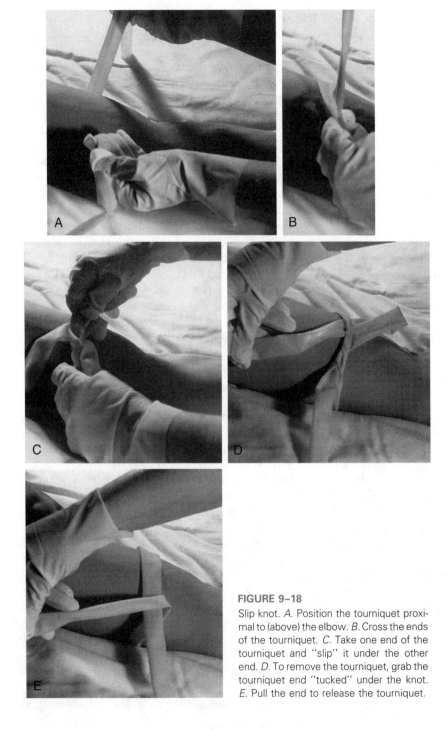

FIGURE 9–18

Slip knot. *A.* Position the tourniquet proximal to (above) the elbow. *B.* Cross the ends of the tourniquet. *C.* Take one end of the tourniquet and "slip" it under the other end. *D.* To remove the tourniquet, grab the tourniquet end "tucked" under the knot. *E.* Pull the end to release the tourniquet.

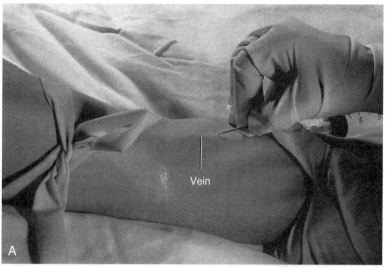

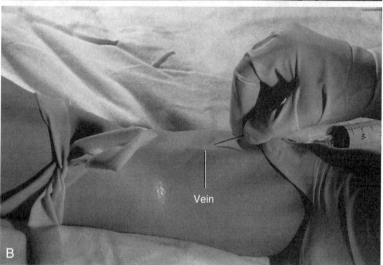

FIGURE 9–19
A. Direct method of venipuncture. Note the needle position is over the vein. *B.* Indirect venipuncture method, in which the needle position is lateral to the vein.

is that in the indirect method the needle is positioned about ¼ inch below and to the lateral side of the vein. The thumb of the nondominant hand pulls the skin taut. Using the dominant hand, the needle is positioned, bevel up, making a 45-degree angle with the skin and is inserted through the skin. Once in the skin, the needle is aimed medially, toward the vein, the angle of the needle is decreased (so that it is almost parallel with the skin), and the needle is inserted into the vein. Needle location is verified with a dark red back flow of blood. After the needle is in the proper position, the appropriate equipment, i.e., IV tubing, is attached.

If an intracatheter is employed, the usual puncture technique is used. After verifying that the needle is in the vein, the catheter and needle are disengaged and the catheter is advanced in the vein. Disengaging the catheter and needle prevents the needle from further puncturing the vein while the catheter is advanced in the vein. When the catheter is in the proper position, the needle is removed from the catheter and the appropriate device, i.e., syringe, is attached.

Regardless of the needle used, once in the vein, it is taped to prevent needle movement within the vein or dislodging out of the vein. There are several different taping methods. Generally, the hospital has its own protocol regarding the taping method of choice. Two common methods are the H method (Fig. 9–20) and the chevron method (Fig. 9–21).

After the medication has been injected, the needle is removed. This is done after carefully removing the tape from the needle. Place a clean gauze over the puncture site. While applying firm pressure to the site with the gauze, remove the needle. Apply pressure until the bleeding has stopped. Bandage the puncture site.

As with all procedures involving the potential for blood or fluid contact, the technologist is advised to follow the proper protective blood/fluid protocol, i.e., wear gloves, wear goggles, and properly dispose of needles.

DIRECT INTRAVENOUS BOLUS INJECTION

Because bolus injections are given in a short period of time (within minutes), a larger (small-gauge in the range of 18–20) needle is preferred. Also, a large vein is recommended for a bolus injection. The most common veins used are the median basilic and median cephalic veins, located in the antecubital area. However, it should be noted that if the needle is going to be in the patient for any length of time, an arm board or other device should be used to stabilize the elbow and prevent it from bending, which could cause injury to the patient.

After the technologist has performed the usual preprocedural care and has located the puncture site, the area is exposed and a bedsaver is placed under the site. A tourniquet is applied 6–8 inches proximal to the puncture site. When the vein is distended, it is ready for puncture. Either the direct or the indirect method of needle puncture (see earlier) may be used. When the puncture is complete, the needle is secured to the patient (see earlier) and the appropriate equipment is attached. After the medication has been administered, the needle is removed and disposed of properly (see earlier).

CONTINUOUS INFUSION INJECTION

The continuous infusion (Fig. 9–22) method employs an infusion bottle (usually for contrast medium), IV tubing, IV pole, and needle as well as the normal IV equipment, e.g., tourniquet. In this method, open the infusion bottle and remove

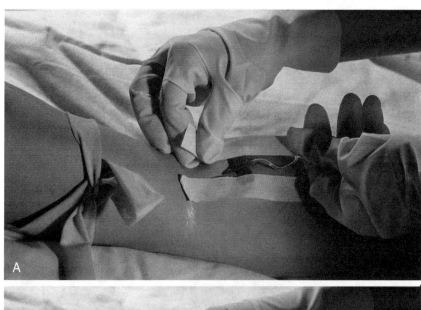

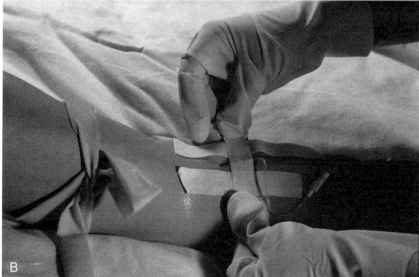

FIGURE 9–20
H method of taping a butterfly needle. *A.* Tape each wing of the needle. *B.* Place another tape perpendicular to tape over the wings and covering the wings.

Illustration continued on following page

the cap on the spike of the IV tubing. Close the clamp on the IV tubing. Insert the spike on the IV tubing into the rubber stopper of the infusion bottle. Hang the bottle upside-down on the IV pole and squeeze the drip chamber until it is half full. Attach the needle to the IV tubing. Allow the fluid in the bottle to flow

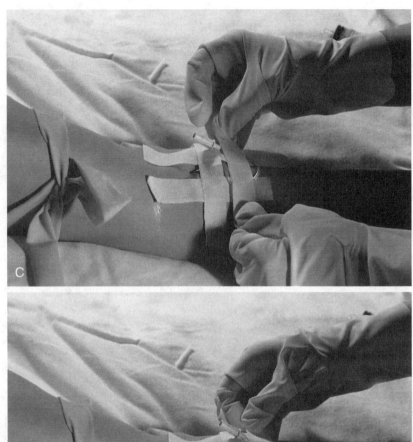

FIGURE 9–20 (*Continued*)
C. Loosely loop the tubing and tape it over the wings. *D.* On another tape, write the date and time the needle was inserted and initial. Put this tape over the tubing tape.

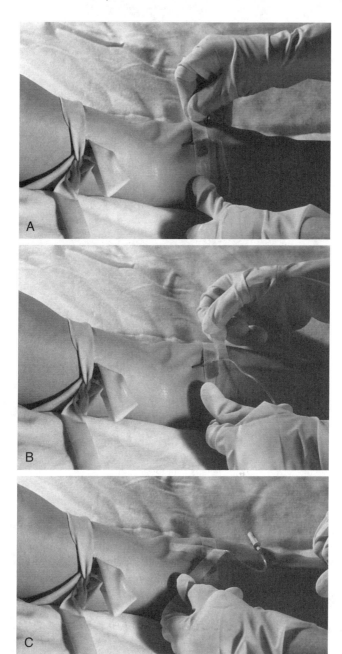

FIGURE 9–21

Chevron taping method. *A.* Place a tape across the needle. *B.* Place a tape under the needle with the adhesive side upward. *C.* Cross each end of the tape over the needle to the opposite side.

Illustration continued on following page

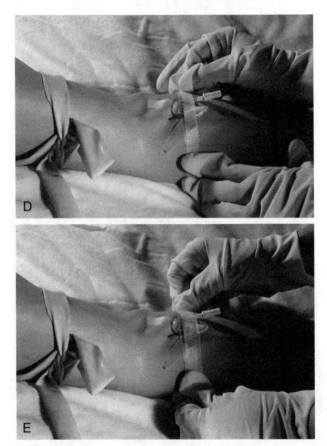

FIGURE 9–21 (*Continued*)
D. Loosely loop the tubing and put the tape over the tubing. *E.* On another tape, write the date and time the needle was inserted and initial. Put this tape over the tubing and attach it to the patient.

through the tubing and needle. Insert the needle and secure it to the patient using the techniques mentioned earlier. Adjust the drip rate and administer the medication to the patient. When all the medication has been administered, remove the needle (see earlier) and dispose of all equipment using proper protocol and safety procedures identified by the institution.

ADDING MEDICATION THROUGH AN ESTABLISHED LINE

Sometimes patients already have an IV line in a vein. It is possible to inject contrast medium through these lines. However, prior to injecting any medication into a line that might contain residue of another medication, the technologist should check with the pharmacist to verify that the drugs are compatible (see Chapter 8, Imaging Pharmaceutical Compatibility).

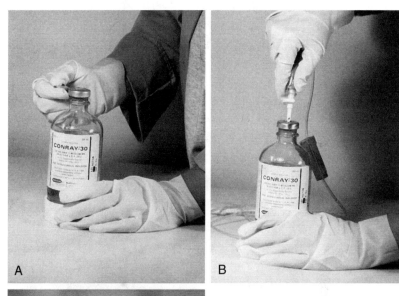

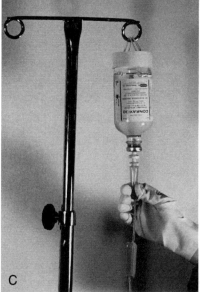

FIGURE 9-22

Continuous infusion injection. *A.* Open the bottle. *B.* Remove the cap from the spike of the intravenous tubing and insert the spike into the bottle. *C.* Hang the bottle upside down on the intravenous (IV) pole and squeeze the drip chamber.

Illustration continued on following page

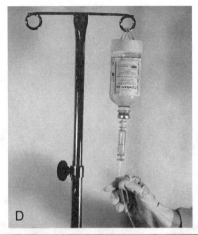

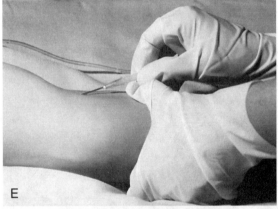

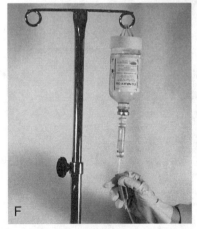

FIGURE 9–22 (*Continued*)
D. Open the clamp on the intravenous tubing to fill the tube. *E.* Attach the needle to the tubing and insert it in the patient. *F.* Use the clamp to adjust the flow rate.

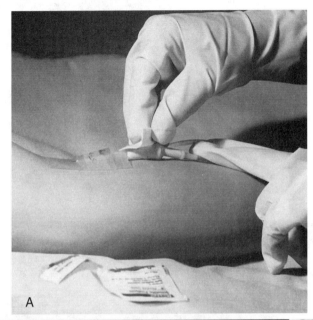

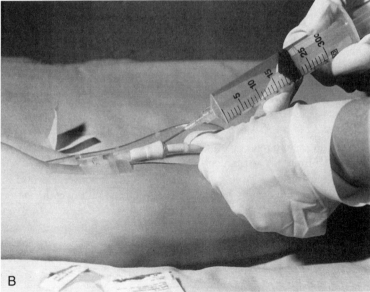

FIGURE 9–23

Injecting through intravenous tubing. *A.* Clean the port. *B.* Insert the needle in the port, and withdraw the plunger to ensure the needle is in the vein.

Illustration continued on following page

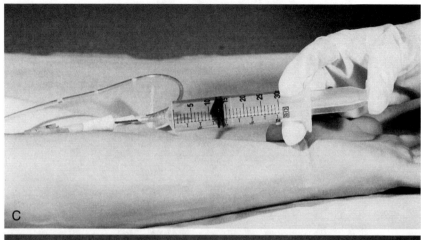

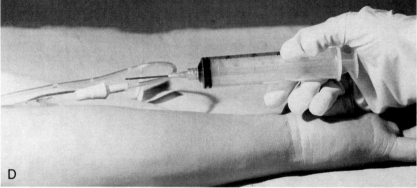

FIGURE 9-23 (*Continued*)
C. Inject the medication. *D.* Remove the needle from the port and readjust the flow rate.

If it is acceptable to inject medication through the established line, close the clamp on the IV tubing. Use an alcohol swab to clean the port on the IV tubing (Fig. 9–23A) and insert a large-gauge needle into the port (see Fig. 9–23B). Withdraw the plunger to ensure that the needle is in the vein. Inject the medication through the port (see Fig. 9–23C). The port may be flushed with 1–2 ml of saline before and after any medication injection. Remove the needle from the port (see Fig. 9–23D) and reopen the clamp on the IV tubing and adjust it to the proper flow rate.

COMPLICATIONS ASSOCIATED WITH INTRAVENOUS INJECTION

Intravenous injection is not without complications. Besides adverse reaction to the medication administered, among the complications are infiltration, infection, circulatory problems, embolism, and phlebitis.

Infiltration occurs when the medication enters the surrounding tissue instead of the vein. Some common symptoms noted with infiltration are swelling, pain, and redness around the puncture site. The most common cause of infiltration is displacement of the needle. If infiltration occurs, the infusion should be stopped immediately and the IV equipment removed. Apply ice (if infiltration is less than 30 minutes old) or warm wet compresses (if the infiltration is more than 30 minutes old). Restart the infusion in another site.

Infection can occur at the puncture site. It is characterized by swelling, soreness, redness, and burning along the vein. Infection is often preventable and is caused by poor aseptic technique or contamination. If infection occurs, the IV line should be discontinued and restarted in another site. Warm compresses may be applied to the infection site. The physician should be notified and the patient checked to determine whether drugs are needed to counteract the infection.

Sometimes too much fluid is given to the patient or the fluid is delivered too rapidly. This may cause circulatory problems, manifested as a decrease in blood pressure, dilation of the veins, rapid breathing, shortness of breath, and wide variance between fluid intake and urine output. If these symptoms occur, the physician should be notified. It is recommended that the infusion be slowed, the patient kept warm, the head elevated, and the vital signs monitored.

Phlebitis is an inflammation of the veins. Possible causes of phlebitis from infusion include irritation of the vein by the medication, injury to the vein by the needle, or clot formation caused by the needle or catheter. Symptoms include sore veins, decreased blood flow, edema, and warm skin above the veins. If phlebitis occurs, the infusion should be discontinued and started in another site. Warm compresses can be applied to the involved areas. The physician should be notified.

BIBLIOGRAPHY

Akesson, EJ, Loeb, JA, and Wilson-Pauwel, L: Thompson's core textbook of anatomy, 2nd edition. JB Lippincott, Philadelphia, 1990.

Channell, SR: Manual for IV therapy procedures, 2nd edition. Medical Economics Books, Oradell, NJ, 1985.

Don, BR, Cheitlin, M, Christiansen, M, et al: Pseudohyperkalemia caused by fist clenching during phlebotomy. N Engl J Med 322(18):1290, 1990.

Edmunds, MW: Introduction to clinical pharmacology. Mosby-Year Book, St. Louis, 1991.

Ehrlich, RA, and McCloskey, ED: Patient care in radiography, 4th edition. Mosby-Year Book, St. Louis, 1993.

Hahn, AB, Oestreich, SJK, and Barkin, RL: Mosby's pharmacology in nursing, 16th edition. CV Mosby, St. Louis, 1986.

Plumer, AL: Principles and practice of IV therapy, 3rd edition. Little, Brown, Boston, 1982.

Robinson, J, editorial director: Managing I.V. therapy. Nursing photobook. Intermed Communications, Inc., Horsham, PA, 1981.

Scherer, JC: Introductory clinical pharmacology, 3rd edition. JB Lippincott, Philadelphia, 1987.

Spencer, RT: Clinical pharmacology and nursing management, 3rd edition. JB Lippincott, Philadelphia, 1989.

Torres, LS: Basic medical techniques and patient care for radiologic technologists, 4th edition. JB Lippincott, Philadelphia, 1993.

Williams, BR, and Baer, CL: Essentials of clinical pharmacology in nursing. Springhouse Corporation, Springhouse, PA, 1992.

Documentation

10

INTRODUCTION

Proper record keeping is essential for appropriate assessment and treatment of the patient. It is also the primary legal documentation of care given to the patient. The hospital or other health care facility is the owner and "keeper" of the patient's records. The length of time a chart is kept is usually defined by state statute. For example, some states require that information be kept on a child until the person reaches the age of majority, usually defined as 18 years of age.

Access to records should be limited to those caring for the patient, those who are legally responsible for the patient, or those identified by law, e.g., in the case of a summons. Also, medical personnel should access only those areas of the record that are relevant to proper performance of their duties.

The type of records kept is usually identified by state laws and hospital policy manuals. These policies should include documentation guidelines such as standards of practice, protocols, and acceptable abbreviations. Some facilities require documentation of the procedure even if the standard protocol was followed, whereas other institutions require that only any variances from the standard procedure be documented. Although the number and type of standards vary among states and institutions, several types of records are standard.

The record keeping process for nurses, physicians, and some other health care professionals tend to have more literature written regarding the proper procedures and methods used for documenting events. Unfortunately, imaging personnel, especially at the technologist's level, tend to be poorly educated in proper documentation procedures. One reason for the lack of standards for imaging personnel may be attributed to the fact that few, if any, patient charts have a form or place to allow the technologist to write comments. Conversely, it is common for the patient's chart to have sections for nurses' notes, physicians' comments, laboratory reports, etc. The tendency is for imaging personnel to record the patient's information on the examination requisition. However, the facility must have a policy regarding the handling of such information. For example, normally, when the patient is discharged, all records are kept in a central location within the institution. However, few facilities require that the imaging department send its records, e.g., comments on requisitions, to the medical records department.

This chapter discusses forms that should be used as part of record keeping relative to the administration of pharmaceuticals in an imaging department. It should be noted that the institution must have a written policy regarding the procedure and the use of any form. For example, a policy might be written regarding the forwarding of a copy of an informed consent form to the medical records department or placed in the patient's chart.

INFORMED CONSENT

Prior to the introduction of any pharmaceutical, the patient should be informed about the procedure, including any medications that must be used. The information should be verbally explained to the patient by the physician in a language the patient understands. After the physician has answered any questions the patient may have about the procedure, a written informed consent document is signed by the patient and by an unbiased person (a person who has no interest in the outcome of the procedure), e.g., a chaplain. Chapter 7, Preventive Care and Emergency Response to Contrast Medium Reactions, contains information about the specific elements of informed consent. Refer to Table 7–1 of that chapter for a sample informed consent document.

Because the technologist is involved in the procedure, it is important that the technologist does *not* witness (sign) the patient's signature on the informed consent document. The technologist's involvement in the procedure makes him or her a subjective or prejudiced witness. Also, the technologist should *not* be the individual advising the patient of the procedure. The primary task of the technologist regarding the informed consent is to review the patient's records to ensure that informed consent has been obtained and that the proper signatures appear on the document. An unsigned informed consent document does not substantiate that the patient either was informed or consented to the procedure. If the informed consent form is unsigned, the examination should be postponed until the procedure has been explained to the patient and the proper signatures have been obtained.

PROCEDURE DATA FORM

After the procedure begins, a form should be available to record information about the procedure. This document is known as the Procedure Data Form (Fig. 10–1). The document contains demographic information, the patient's allergy history, radiograph count and technical factors, information on the type of medications and contrast media administered, catheterization method, vital signs, laboratory results, and a section for instructions or comments.

The demographic profile is basic information about the patient such as name, age, and sex. It is important to document all allergies of the patient. The radiograph count and technical factors are helpful in calculating the amount of radiation exposure the patient might have received. It is important to record all radiographs taken, even if they were repeated. A note should be made regarding repeat radiographs because these are disposed of and do not become a part of the patient's record. For example, if the Procedure Data Form identified that five radiographs were taken, but only four are in the patient's folder, there should be documentation explaining the location of the fifth radiograph, e.g., it was disposed of because it was undiagnostic (contained static) and needed to be repeated. A record should be kept of all the pharmaceuticals administered (including contrast media). At a minimum, this information should identify the name of the medication, route of administration, the quantity administered, the time of administration, and the name of the person who administered the medication. For procedures requiring the patient to be catheterized, a record is kept of the side(s) catheterized, vessel, catheter size, catheter type, and approach (e.g., translumbar). A record of the patient's vital signs is also documented. The vital signs section of Figure 10–1 is designed to measure the pre- and postprocedural readings; however, the form can be edited to include any reading obtained during the procedure. Laboratory results are recorded in the appropriate place on the procedure form. The laboratory procedures listed in Figure 10–1 are the areas of prime concern for most imaging procedures; additional laboratory results can be added to the form. The section identified as comments or instructions is useful in documenting any event that is outside the standard procedure, e.g., reaction to contrast medium.

COMPLICATION OR INCIDENT REPORT

In the rare instance of a complication, a report should be completed documenting the adverse reaction and the treatment or response administered. The form is usually entitled Complication or Incident Report (Fig. 10–2). It should document the persons present at the time of the occurrence and the personnel completing the report. It is important to follow up on any complication that may occur. Thus, the form should also contain a section to document the follow-up care. As always, the form should also contain a section for comments.

Many institutions also have a form used to assess the performance of the health care team. This form is often called a Risk Management Form (Fig. 10–3). The primary objective is to assess the events that occurred to determine what, if anything, should be done to improve the health care team's response for any future complication. One of the potential problems of the form is that it documents errors that might have occurred. These errors may be used against the facility in a lawsuit. The risk of documenting errors should not deter the institution from having a Risk Management Form. The form is necessary to improve care and help document the care provided for accreditation purposes. Also, historically, health care providers are liable when negligence, assault, battery, or false imprisonment can be proven. Thus, unless the documented error falls into one of these categories, the team would probably be found innocent of any medical malpractice.

CHARTING

If the policy of the institution is for the technologist to write the information discussed earlier in the patient's chart, the technologist must input the information in a concise, accurate, objective, and complete manner. Because few technologists have any education on documentation, this section is dedicated to providing some suggestions as to charting techniques.

It is important to be concise in describing events. Embellishing the event should be avoided. All the information should accurately reflect the events that

JOHN SMITH HOSPITAL

IMAGING DEPARTMENT

Patient's Name _____ Age _____ Sex _____ DOB _____

Medical Records No: _____ Date _____ Location _____

Procedure _____ Requesting Dr: _____ Date of order _____

SPECIAL INSTRUCTIONS

1. _____

2. _____

3. _____

ALLERGY HISTORY

Source: _____ Patient   _____ Records   _____ Other

Type(s) _____

CHECKLIST	YES	NO	N/A	STATISTICS		RADIOGRAPHY	RADIOGRAPH COUNT DIGITAL	DUPLICATING
Patient identified	__	__	__	Time in	_____	8 × 10	_____ _____	_____
Procedure identified	__	__	__	Exam time	_____	9 × 9	_____ _____	_____
Pregnancy status	__	__	__	Time out	_____	7 × 17	_____ _____	_____
Informed consent	__	__	__	Fluoro time	_____	10 × 12	_____ _____	_____
Exam completion	__	__	__	Radiologist	_____	11 × 14	_____ _____	_____
Exam rescheduled	__	__	__	Technologist	_____	14 × 14	_____ _____	_____
Discharge instructions	__	__	__	Technologist	_____	14 × 17	_____ _____	_____
Condition Unchanged	__	__	__	Other	_____	_____	_____ _____	_____

FIGURE 10–1

Sample Procedure Data Form. (The form is reprinted with permission from Tortorici, MR, and Apfel, PJ: Advanced radiographic and angiographic procedures with an introduction to specialized imaging. FA Davis, Philadelphia, 1995. The figure of the hand on the form is reprinted with permission from Shila, RC: Manual for IV therapy procedures, 2nd ed. PMIC, Los Angeles, 1985. The figure of the arm on the form is reprinted with permission from Plumer, AC: Principles and practices of intravenous therapy, 3rd edition. Little, Brown, Boston, 1982.)

Illustration continued on facing page

DISPOSITION			SKIN PREP		TECHNICAL FACTORS			
LOCATION	TO	FROM	Area	_____ Type of Filming	mA	Time	kVp	
Inpatient	_____	_____	Shave prep	_____ POSITION/RUN 1	___	___	___	___
Outpatient	_____	_____	Antiseptic scrub	_____ POSITION/RUN 2	___	___	___	___
Outpatient surgery	_____	_____	By: _____	_____ POSITION/RUN 3	___	___	___	___
ER	_____	_____	**ANESTHETIC**	_____ POSITION/RUN 4	___	___	___	___
ICU	_____	_____	Type	_____ POSITION/RUN 5	___	___	___	___
Surgery	_____	_____	Method of Adm.	_____ POSITION/RUN 6	___	___	___	___
Other	_____	_____	Adm. By:	_____ POSITION/RUN 7	___	___	___	___

_____ _____ _____

CATHETERIZATION METHOD

MODE OF TRANSPORTATION			SIDE	VESSEL	CATHETER SIZE	CATHETER TYPE	TYPE OF APPROACH
	TO	FROM	1. _____	_____	_____	_____	_____
Ambulatory	_____	_____	2. _____	_____	_____	_____	_____

FIGURE 10–1 (*Continued*)
Illustration continued on following page

occurred. Although brevity is encouraged, it is important that the information be complete. Subjective terms should be avoided. Examples of common subjective wording include terms such as "small," "large," and "The patient was drunk." Relating facts is the easiest way to avoid subjectivity. For example, a subjective statement might be "Several needle punctures had to be made because the patient was a drug addict." Unless the patient admitted to being an intravenous drug user who injected the drugs at the site the technologist was trying to puncture, this statement is subjective. However, it is possible to write objective observable data such as "The right basilic vein was very movable" or "There were numerous small scars around the needle entry site" (the exact location of the site would have to be identified in a previous statement or marked on a diagram). These are observable items that can be documented without presenting a subjective opinion about the patient.

Figure 10–1, a Procedure Data Form, is an example of one form that can be used for documenting procedural events. It is helpful to have the form contain diagrams of the veins and arteries, which can be used to document injection sites. The diagrams allow the user to place an "X" over the correct location of the needle entry site and an "O" over any area that underwent an unsuccessful puncture attempt. It is also important to identify whether the site is on the right or left side of the patient's body. The number of diagrams on the form may vary.

(*Text continued on page 152*)

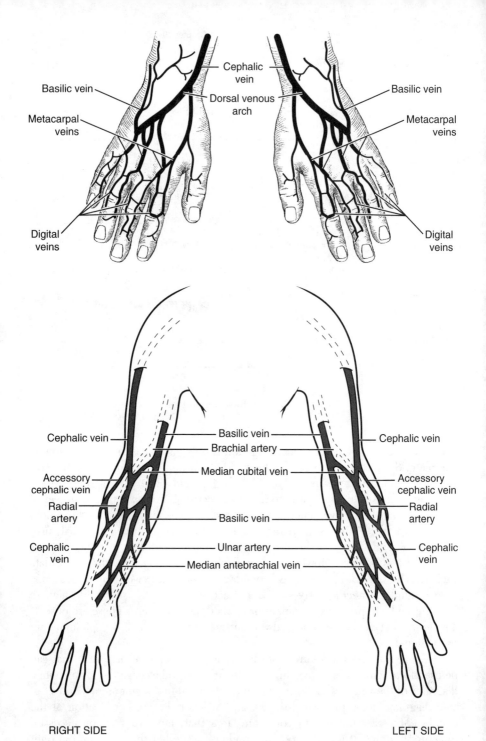

Cephalic vein

Basilic vein

Dorsal venous arch

Metacarpal veins

Digital veins

Cephalic vein

Accessory cephalic vein

Radial artery

Cephalic vein

Basilic vein

Brachial artery

Median cubital vein

Basilic vein

Ulnar artery

Median antebrachial vein

Cephalic vein

Accessory cephalic vein

Radial artery

Cephalic vein

RIGHT SIDE

LEFT SIDE

FIGURE 10–1 (*Continued*)

Illustration continued on facing page

CONTRAST MEDIA

ROUTE   TYPE   AMOUNT TIME ADMINISTERED   BY

1. _____ _____ _____ _____ _____

2. _____ _____ _____ _____ _____

3. _____ _____ _____ _____ _____

4. _____ _____ _____ _____ _____

            TOTAL _____

MEDICINE ADMINISTRATION RECORD

TYPE   ROUTE   AMOUNT TIME   BY

1. _____ _____ _____ _____ _____

2. _____ _____ _____ _____ _____

3. _____ _____ _____ _____ _____

4. _____ _____ _____ _____ _____

5. _____ _____ _____ _____ _____

6. _____ _____ _____ _____ _____

INSTRUCTIONS AND/OR COMMENTS

_____

_____

_____

_____

_____

_____

_____

RADIOLOGIST _____

FIGURE 10-1 (*Continued*)

COMPLICATION OR INCIDENT REPORT

Patient _____

Date of emergency _____

Date of evaluation _____

Personnel present and evaluating:

_____

_____

_____

Person(s) completing the incident report.

_____

_____

_____

Briefly describe the complication or incident that occurred.

_____

_____

_____

Summarize the treatment that was administered.

_____

_____

_____

Summarize the follow-up treatment that occurred.

_____

_____

_____

Additional remarks:

_____

_____

_____

FIGURE 10–2
Sample Complication/Incident Report Form. (From Tortorici, MR, and Apfel, PJ: Advanced radiographic and angiographic procedures with an introduction to specialized imaging. FA Davis, Philadelphia, 1995.)

RISK MANAGEMENT SURVEY

Patient _____

Date of emergency _____ Date of evaluation _____

Personnel present and evaluating:

_____

_____

Person(s) completing the incident report.

_____

_____

Was needed equipment readily available? If not, what was missing?

_____

_____

Did personnel present do what was required of them? Did they initiate treatment of their own?

_____

_____

_____

Did auxiliary personnel (e.g., ECG) respond promptly?

_____

_____

_____

What could have been done differently for a more effective and efficient emergency procedure?

_____

_____

_____

Additional remarks:

_____

_____

_____

FIGURE 10–3
Sample Risk Management Form. (From Tortorici, MR, and Apfel, PJ: Advanced radiographic and angiographic procedures with an introduction to specialized imaging. FA Davis, Philadelphia, 1995.)

One design can contain vascular diagrams of sections of the body that are the most common sites for injections, e.g., arm, hand, and that allow the user to identify whether the diagram represents the left or right side. Another may have two full body diagrams of the primary areas of vascular injection sites, one for veins and one for arteries. It is helpful if the form has a duplicate set of diagrams. This is beneficial when an unsuccessful attempt is made on the right side, but a successful injection is made on the left side. Thus, one diagram can be used for identifying the unsuccessful attempts ("O") and the other for the successful attempt ("X"). If the form contains only one venous diagram of the arm, it becomes difficult to demonstrate bilateral injection attempts.

Several precautions should be adhered to when charting. These include:

1. Make entries in the order of occurrence
2. Record the date of the event
3. Note the time of the event
4. Verify that the document refers to the correct patient
5. Sign the entry
6. Use only abbreviations on the institution's approved list
7. Record events only after they have occurred
8. Chart only events in which you were directly involved
9. If you make an error, draw a single line through the error, so the words are still readable; then correct the error and initial it
10. Write in pen
11. Use only forms that are approved by the hospital
12. Record items as soon as possible after they occur
13. Don't add, delete, or otherwise change previously written notes; rather, provide an addendum
14. State the facts, not opinions

BIBLIOGRAPHY

Read, AB: Documentation. RT Image 5(32):6, August 10, 1992.

Edmunds, MW: Introduction to clinical pharmacology. Mosby-Year Book, St. Louis, 1991.

Hahn, AB, Oestreich, SJK, Barkin, RL, et al: Mosby's pharmacology in nursing, 16th edition. CV Mosby, St. Louis, 1986.

Obergfell, AM: Medical legal implications. *In* Tortorici, MR, and Apfel, PJ: Advanced radiographic and angiographic procedures with an introduction to specialized imaging. FA Davis, Philadelphia, 1995.

Spencer, RT, Nichols, LW, Lipkin, GB, et al: Clinical pharmacology and nursing management, 3rd edition. JB Lippincott, Philadelphia, 1989.

Williams, BR, and Baer, CL: Essentials of clinical pharmacology in nursing. Springhouse Corporation, Springhouse, PA, 1990.

Index

Note: Page numbers in *italics* refer to illustrations; page numbers followed by (t) refer to tables.